BREAKAWAY

The International Medical Graduate's Guide to Alternative Careers

NICOLE GUEVARA, MD, MSHI, CPHIMS

First published by Ultimate World Publishing 2021
Copyright © 2021 Nicole Guevara

ISBN

Paperback: 978-1-922714-47-3
Ebook: 978-1-922597-62-5

Nicole Guevara has asserted her rights under the Copyright, Designs and Patents Act 1988 to be identified as the author of this work. The information in this book is based on the author's experiences and opinions. The publisher specifically disclaims responsibility for any adverse consequences which may result from use of the information contained herein. Permission to use information has been sought by the author. Any breaches will be rectified in further editions of the book.

All rights reserved. No part of this publication may be reproduced, stored in or introduced into a retrieval system, or transmitted in any form, or by any means (electronic, mechanical, photocopying, recording or otherwise) without the prior written permission of the author. Any person who does any unauthorized act in relation to this publication may be liable to criminal prosecution and civil claims for damages. Enquiries should be made through the publisher.

Cover design: Ultimate World Publishing
Layout and typesetting: Ultimate World Publishing
Editor: Emily Riches
Cover photo: Sergey Nivens-Shutterstock.com

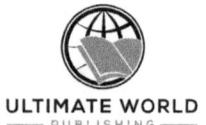

Ultimate World Publishing
Diamond Creek,
Victoria Australia 3089
www.writeabook.com.au

Testimonials

"One of the most insightful and creative minds I have encountered in 20 years of working in healthcare. A leader among her peers, whose transformative thought processes provide a spark to patients and providers alike. An innovator who has a drive to make an indelible improvement to our healthcare delivery system."

Brian A. White, NP

"Once a doctor, forever a life dedicated in service to others. *Breakaway* is a testament to Nicole's journey, gaining wisdom through her own challenges, sharing her insight, and undoubtedly inspiring others. It is a shining beacon for those looking to reimagine a life outside of medicine."

Camille Lachica, BSN, CV-BC, CDP
Interim Nursing Director, Neuroscience
Robert Wood Johnson University Medical Center

"Nicole's book *Breakaway* will help you navigate the difficult waters that is the transition from one career path to another. Her concise, clear, and honest advice is what makes the book so appealing and easy to read. On a personal note, working with Nicole is a pleasure. Her depth of knowledge in the healthcare field, willingness to collaborate, and most importantly her commitment to excellence makes her an unparalleled colleague. Her personal success shows in her work. *Breakaway* will be worth your time."

Migdalia Pino
Contracts Manager

"Nicole has an extreme breadth of knowledge of the healthcare field and a profound interest in expanding her skill set. Her level of expertise and understanding of managed care programs and their impact on the health and wellness of patients is unparalleled. She has a keen awareness of the importance of health informatics and its influence on the future of healthcare and is well-equipped with the tools and knowledge needed to educate and mentor those seeking to improve the healthcare system."

Dr. Monica R. Rider
Board Certified Family Physician
CMO of an FQHC

"Health service is a complicated mix of old and new ideas and/or processes. Nicole brings her passion for healthy outcomes for patients and fresh innovative ideas to each area she invests in. She has the medical knowledge that is the foundation of health services and, coupled with her analytical analysis, she transforms old processes into more efficient data-driven decisions. Her insightful personality allows her to uncover new and dynamic avenues of improvement opportunities. She possesses a courageous spirit that leads her to explore the multifaceted world of health care."

Raven Chen
Data Analyst Manager

"No matter the magnitude of the question or how complex the problem, Nicole always manages to find the answer. Given her vast experience of the healthcare industry, there is no doubt I would turn to her for guidance. She can analyze any situation from different points, based on her experience, in order to produce results – not to mention her ability to back up each solution with data. She is a woman who is always thinking ahead to ensure the data fits the solution. Nicole is not only intelligent, she is also compassionate and willing to help anyone in need."

Bianca Perez
Senior Patient Engagement Specialist

"I am so glad Nicole wrote this book! As an IMG myself, having the guidance and resources from Nicole about alternatives in applying medical skills and knowledge is a godsend. Having a mentor who went through the same processes gave me a boost of confidence that I will be able to recalibrate and find my purpose."

Dr. Fiona Avry

In loving memory of my superman dad (Doc Alex) who inspired me
to be fearless and taught me the essence of giving.

For my loving family – my mom (Doc Mergie), my brother (Patrick),
my sister (Doc Angel), and my brother-in-law (Doc Jake) – who taught me
the power of hope and encouraged me to aspire without limit.

Contents

Testimonials 3
Introduction 9

Thoughts

    Chapter 1: Realize Your Breakthrough and Get Ready to Break Away 15
    Chapter 2: Refocus Your Vision and Reinvent Your Perspective 21
    Chapter 3: Redevelop a Growth Mindset and Restructure Your Neurons. 27

Knowledge

    Chapter 4: Burnout Counselor 33
    Chapter 5: Certified Life Coach and Cancer Coach 41
    Chapter 6: Clinical Content Manager 51
    Chapter 7: Entrepreneur 57
    Chapter 8: Global Health Advisor 67
    Chapter 9: Health Informatics Specialist 75
    Chapter 10: Health Insurance Advisor 83
    Chapter 11: Home Health Care Continuum 91
    Chapter 12: Medical Educator 101
    Chapter 13: Medical Reviewer 109
    Chapter 14: Medical Science Liaison 117
    Chapter 15: Medical Scientist 125
    Chapter 16: Pharmaceutical Ethics and Compliance Continuum 133
    Chapter 17: Planetary Doctor 141
    Chapter 18: Professor 149
    Chapter 19: Quality Coordinator 157
    Chapter 20: Ship Physician 165

Action
- Chapter 21: Sharpen Your Knowledge 173
- Chapter 22: Select Your Mentors 177
- Chapter 23: Strengthen Your Network. 181

References 185
Testimonials (continued) 205
Acknowledgments 207
About the Author. 209

Introduction

"If you cannot find the resource you're looking for, create it."
– **Nicole Guevara**

Are you a medical graduate who wants to pursue an alternative career from traditional medicine? Are you lost in your career transition and do not know where to start? Are you jumping from one job to another, not gaining any traction with a valuable career? Then this book is for you. My objective is to provide a powerful guide to help you pivot from medicine.

The title *Breakaway* signifies an international medical graduate's (IMG) career transition. It amplifies the courage, determination, perseverance, hard work, sweat, and tears an IMG experiences as he/she transitions from a medical path to an unknown direction. It highlights the trials, tribulations, challenges, victories, and rewards an IMG undergoes as he/she "breaks away" from medicine.

My Story

Let me humbly begin by sharing my story – my raw and honest experience. I am an international medical graduate who graduated with my Doctor of Medicine degree from West Visayas State University College of Medicine (WVSU-COM) in Iloilo City, Philippines in 2012. My family immigrated to the US from the Philippines when I was 13 years old, settling in Clearwater, Florida. After receiving my bachelor's degree from the University of Florida in global health issues, my intention was to receive a Master of Public Health (MPH) degree and work for the World Health Organization (WHO) organizing community development and health programs. I saw myself as an idealistic trailblazer serving third world countries in program management and saving lives from infectious and tropical diseases such as dengue and malaria.

After a month-long family vacation to our home city in the Philippines, I realized medical school might be a better path to realizing my future aspirations. I never considered US medical schools because, as a dual citizen of the US and the Philippines, I could attend a Philippine medical school for a fraction of the cost, be exempt from pre-requisite courses, and receive critical clinical experience in a third world county, preparing me for a job with the WHO.

Spending considerable time serving rural communities during my 4th year clinical clerkships, I got a taste of what my daily future life would be. Outdoor cold showers, long days of community health clinic consults without internet access or air conditioning in 90+ degree humid weather, and cooking dinner over an open fire began weighing on me. I realized I was not built for the life I was seeking. I missed hot showers, the comfort of air conditioning, and a consistent internet connection I had taken for granted in the US. The idea of working for the WHO no longer matched my reality. I also missed my family tremendously. So I went back to Florida after medical school graduation.

Back in the US in 2013, I took and failed my USMLE (United States Medical Licensing Examination) Step 1 exam. I also took and failed my USMLE Step 2 Clinical Skills (CS) exam. Disheartened, I fell into depression, grieving and mourning my underachievement. For two years, I navigated through different careers trying to figure out where I belonged. I worked as a caregiver for a home health agency, a patient care technician for a dialysis clinic, and a counselor for a drug rehabilitation facility. I had no goal and doubt overcame me. I wondered whether I was even meant to be in the US.

In 2015, I returned to the Philippines, planning to live there after completing my post-graduate internship training at Manila Doctors Hospital. After a year of clinical rotations, each department nominated a candidate for the Most Outstanding Intern Award which was based on scholarship, leadership, community involvement, and stewardship. In 2016, I received that award as the most outstanding intern for the entire hospital. Thinking I was on the right track, I applied, took, and failed my Philippine Physician Licensure Examination (Philippine medical boards) – twice. Again, I became disheartened and fell into depression and doubt. Again, I grieved and mourned my underachievement. This time, however, I was inclined to do something about it. Every day, I sought refuge in nature, deeply searching my soul for an answer. Then, it dawned on me: I had self-sabotaged. I failed my licensure examinations because I hadn't applied myself wholeheartedly. I never put in the long hours of studying required. In fact, I found every reason not to study. Suddenly, it became clear: I didn't want to be a doctor.

Dumbfounded, this revelation stopped me in my tracks. Both my parents were doctors – my father a surgeon and my mother an anesthesiologist – in the Philippines. I was surrounded by doctors, medical missionaries, hospitals, and patients my entire life and I wanted to become a part of my parents' mission to make the world a better place through medicine. But medicine wasn't for me. I needed my own path. The truth was, my parents never pressured me to become a doctor. They simply advocated for finding a meaningful and fulfilling life. So I strived to follow my dream.

In 2017, I returned to Florida armed with determination and optimism. I spent months in reflection and prayer. I love the humanitarian side of health care, but I am more interested in the business side of the industry, rather than clinical care. I'm also fairly skilled in the area of technology. I began focusing on finding a rewarding career centered around these three interests. In 2018, I started my Master of Science in Health Informatics degree at the University of South Florida. I was a sponge, eager to soak up every bit of knowledge and information I could get my hands on. While in school I worked full-time in a doctor's office learning everything I could about practice management and the business side of the healthcare industry. I worked as a medical assistant, back-office assistant, front desk personnel, referrals coordinator, clinical documentation specialist, and clinical manager for that same office. The humbling nature of doing entry-level, back-office work when I had worked so hard to earn a medical doctorate was uncomfortable. However, this training ground sparked a fervor in me that I was, indeed, capable of running a medical practice.

In 2019, a few months before graduation, I was hired as a Clinical Data Analyst for Florida's largest Federally Qualified Health Center (FQHC) with 15 health centers in the Tampa Bay Area and 80-90 multi-specialty healthcare providers. In 2019, the health centers saw roughly 109,000 patients over 300,000 visits. I was in my element. Two months later, I was promoted to Director of Managed Care and Business Development supervising a team of data analysts. In another seven months I became Director of Performance Outcomes supervising a team of Patient Engagement Specialists and a Medical Reviewer. Presently, I am doing what I love leveraging my knowledge and experience as a full-time healthcare consultant serving large scale healthcare organizations globally.

Lessons From My Story

I learned that it is okay to start from square one. Starting anew did not mean I failed my previous endeavor, it meant there was something better in store for me. It meant I needed to work harder and smarter to achieve something even more amazing. No one can ever take my education and accomplishments away from me. No one can dictate my thoughts and actions. I learned I am the captain of my own ship and in charge of my own destiny. I had to humbly welcome new challenges. As a seed needs darkness in the soil before it sprouts into a beautiful flower, I needed to experience my own darkness. As a plant needs pruning to become strong and healthy, I needed to search my soul for answers. As a grape needs crushing before becoming sweet wine, I needed to experience ultimate disappointment. My story serves as my training ground. The valuable lessons I learned propelled me to my next adventure.

The IMG's Journey

An International Medical Graduate (IMG) is a physician who received his/her medical degree outside of the country where he/she intends to practice. In the United States, the National Residency Matching Program (NRMP) reported that in 2020, there were 12,074 active IMG applicants of which 7,376 (61.1%) matched to their preferred specialty. In 2019, there were 11,949 active IMG applicants of which 7,025 (58.8%) matched.[1] In 2018, there were a total of 12,142 active IMG applicants of which 6,229 (51.3%) matched.[2]

In the NRMP Report for 2018, the active IMG applicants completed numerous work, research, and volunteer experiences. IMGs averaged 5.1 work experiences and 81% participated in more than one work experience. IMGs also averaged 2.25 research experiences and 64.4% conducted more than one study. IMGs averaged 4.1 volunteer experiences and 78.35% had more than one volunteer experience. Furthermore, approximately 2.3% of the active IMG applicants held a PhD degree in addition to a MD degree.[2]

Why have I shared these statistics? I want you to glean how extraordinary IMGs are everywhere. They are researchers, clinicians, academicians, and philanthropists. IMGs are hardworking and dedicated overachievers who comprise a valuable untapped workforce. These statistics uncover stories of personal resilience, resourcefulness, and versatility.

This book will equip IMGs with resources to move into fulfilling careers. It is divided into three sections: Thoughts, Knowledge, and Action. Its main objectives are to renew your thoughts, arm you with knowledge, and motivate your actions.

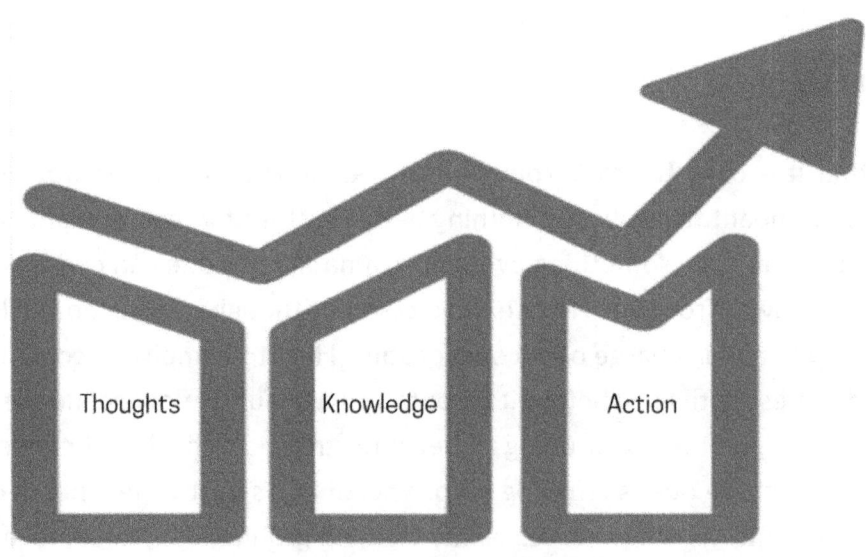

Research of the human brain suggests the average person has approximately 6,000 thoughts a day.[3] How we think dictates how we feel and act toward a stimulus in our life. Our thoughts are cultivated from the reception of information to deciding on what to do with that knowledge. Thoughts influence our beliefs and, ultimately, our actions. They define our plans, experiences, circumstances, and reactions. Fortunately, we have the ability to consciously choose our thoughts. We can choose to think either positively or negatively. Thus, we can increase our joy by thinking of pleasant experiences. In this way, our thoughts become our reality.

The first section of this book emphasizes the importance of aligning thoughts with desires. You will begin with realizing your own breakthrough, refocusing your vision, and reinventing your perspectives. Each chapter highlights exemplary persons in history who have made significant contributions to humanity and illustrates their journey to becoming experts in their fields. By the conclusion of this section, you will be well on your way to redeveloping your growth mindset and restructuring your neurons. You will also receive challenges to create headway for beginning your journey.

The second section will arm you with knowledge of available alternative careers, highlighting interviews with medical doctors around the world who pivoted to non-traditional careers outside of medicine. Each chapter contains an overview, a definition of the profession, a sample case, and the roles and responsibilities of that career. It then progresses to the necessary skills and training needed to succeed, the pros and cons of the career, and future growth potential. Each profession is woven with anecdotes from a professional in that field. Each chapter concludes with a "Now What?" scenario suggesting steps you can take to start that career. Armed with the congruence of thoughts and knowledge, you will be ready to embark on actionable strategies.

Thoughts and knowledge accomplish little without accompanying action. The third section explains how to put ideas to work by suggesting tangible activities that will make you a robust candidate for your chosen career. It tackles the importance of sharpening your knowledge, strengthening your network, and selecting your mentors. Each chapter provides a step-by-step guide to pursuing each activity. By the end of the chapter, you will also receive a challenge to escalate your progress.

CHALLENGE 1:

Now that I have shared my story, it is time to write down your story. This exercise is important because you must outline the truth behind your struggle before the door can be opened for your metamorphoses to occur. Connect with me on any of my social media platforms. Together, we will create a network of IMGs who will pivot/have pivoted to careers outside of medicine. Why? Through these platforms, I will provide the tools and resources you need to leverage your skills.

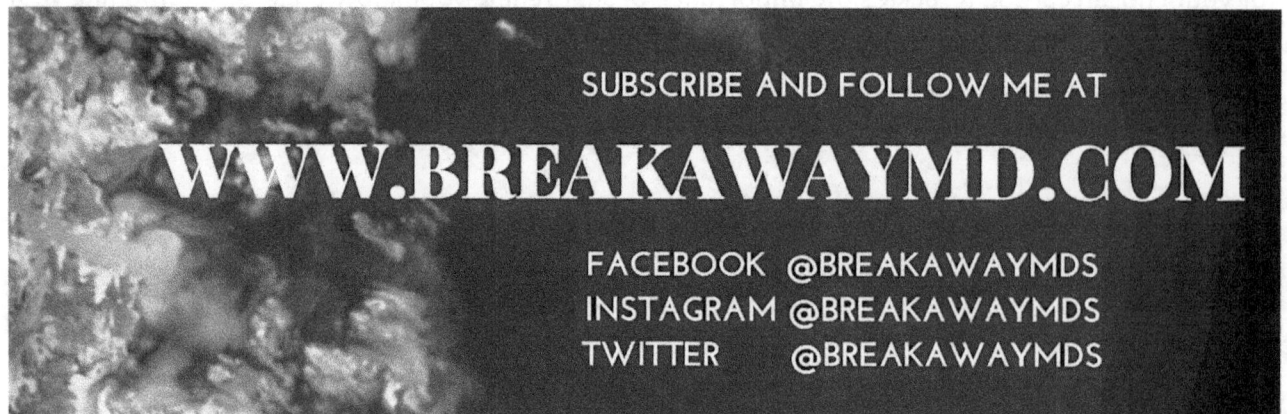

SUBSCRIBE AND FOLLOW ME AT
WWW.BREAKAWAYMD.COM
FACEBOOK @BREAKAWAYMDS
INSTAGRAM @BREAKAWAYMDS
TWITTER   @BREAKAWAYMDS

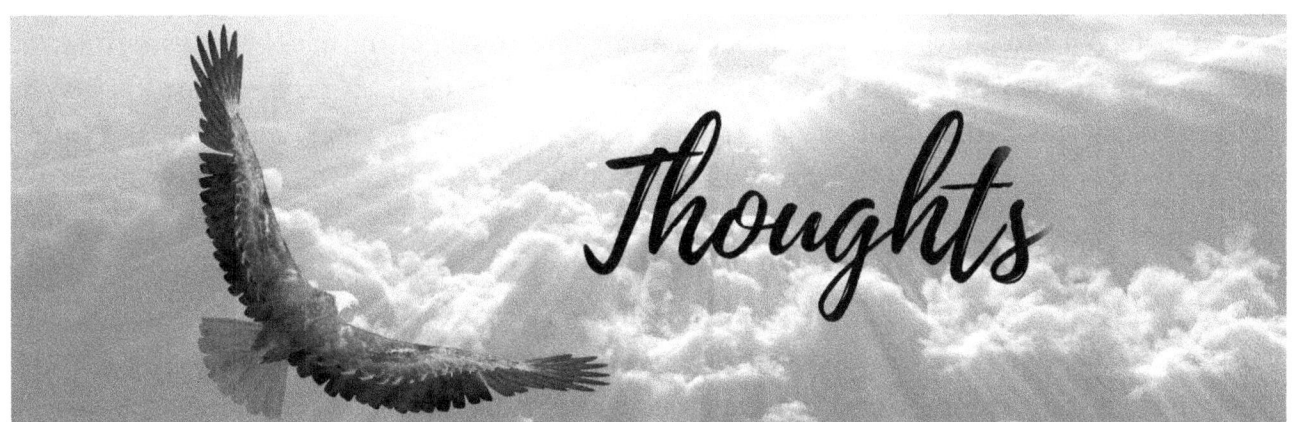

Chapter 1

Realize Your Breakthrough and Get Ready to Break Away

The eagle loves storms. When the skies darken and the clouds gather, the eagle becomes eager. As the storm breaks, the eagle uses strong winds to lift itself higher and higher above the clouds. The storm gives the eagle a chance to glide and rest its wings 10,000 feet above land, while the other birds cower and huddle in tree branches.[4] Are you ready to embrace the storms of your life like the eagle? Neither growth nor development occur in comfort zones. Breaking away from your comfort zone will allow you to discover something new and experience the profound. Rise and soar to new heights. Now is the time to realize your breakthrough and get ready to break away.

A large portion of your life has been dedicated to learning medicine. You studied anatomy and physiology, biochemistry, and parasitology in year one. Do you remember the cadaver dissections? The stench that never left your uniform? Did you ever wish you could take the cranium home for additional study time? You went through surgery, pediatrics, and internal medicine blocks in years two and three. Do you remember taking medical histories and physical examination interviews and practices? How about psychiatric interview practice with your partner? Do you remember the 8-point ophthalmological eye exam?

You lugged 2-to-5-inch medical textbooks from home to school and back home every day. You brought them to the 24-hour coffee shop on the corner or the 24-hour library. You lost track of the sleepless nights you endured and missed countless birthdays, anniversaries, weddings, and special events. You were an avid and exhausted medical student.

Then, you dedicated a portion of your life to healing and saving lives. You completed hospital rotations in years three and four. You wore your first white coat and your first scrubs. You bought your first stethoscope. You experienced a 24-hour duty followed by grand rounds on a rare case. Then, you had your second 24-hour duty, followed by a lengthy morning endorsement. You cleaned and smelled a diabetic foot. You assisted on a below-knee amputation secondary to a non-healing wound secondary to Diabetes Mellitus Type 2. You assisted on an exploratory laparotomy secondary to abdominal trauma. You helped on a laparoscopic appendectomy. You delivered your second 38-week (age of gestation) baby girl to a multigravida via natural birth and your second 39-week (age of gestation) baby boy to a G3P2103 via caesarian section. All this was accomplished in two weeks as an eager senior medical student.

You were then conferred the degree Doctor of Medicine and pledged the Hippocratic Oath, promising to uphold the lofty medical ethic of examining and contemplating your patients' best interests and refraining from doing harm. You vowed to live an exemplary life professionally and personally.[5] You can still uphold this oath, albeit indirectly.

Now, it is time to pivot away from medicine to an alternative career. Medicine knows no boundaries; you should know no limitations. Armed with medical knowledge and prowess, you can work in the fields of health informatics, research, home health nursing, and many more possibilities. You can practice on any healthcare stage. This is your story. This is your life. Realize your breakthrough. Consider the following breakthrough stories.

Smallpox Vaccine Breakthrough in 1776

Smallpox or "speckled monster" plagued human existence since 10,000 BCE during the first agricultural settlements in Africa. The disease was significant in the decline of the Roman Empire during the Plague of Antonine. It was also instrumental in the fall of the Aztec and Incan Empires.[6]

This changed in 1776 with a scientist named Edward Jenner. He hadn't planned on ridding the world of the speckled monster and saving millions of lives. He had no idea he would come to be known as the father of immunology. However, that is exactly what happened. Jenner was curious, meticulous, and skillfully observant. He observed that milkmaids infected with cowpox were never infected with smallpox, although he was not the first scientist to discover the correlation between the two diseases. He also observed that smallpox was transmitted via human-to-human contact. He conducted nationwide research, sending surveys throughout Europe to smallpox survivors searching for proof of his observations.[6]

To test his hypothesis, Jenner found a milkmaid, Ms. Nelm, who had fresh cowpox lesions on her arms and hands. He collected fluid samples from Ms. Nelm's fresh lesions and inoculated an 8-year-old boy with Ms. Nelm's cowpox virus. The boy developed mild fever and discomfort at the inoculation site, but no cowpox disease was produced. A few weeks later, Jenner inoculated the boy with matter from a fresh smallpox lesion, yet he never developed the disease. Strictly speaking, Jenner was not the first to discover vaccination, but he was the first to document the procedure and back it with scientific research and investigation.[6] Thus, Jenner discovered the vaccine for smallpox and systematized the foundations of immunology.

In 1979, 3,000 years after its discovery, Somalia had the last known natural case of the speckled monster. In 1980, the World Health Organization declared smallpox as an eradicated disease after its global smallpox immunization campaign.[7] In 2019, the world celebrated the 40th anniversary of smallpox eradication. WHO Director General Tedros Adhanom Ghebreyesus has classified smallpox as "the only human disease ever eradicated."[8]

Lessons From Edward Jenner

You have a specific set of skills, characteristics, and values that is uniquely yours — a fingerprint driven by your core principles and beliefs. This one-of-a-kind blueprint was created for making a difference, whether in medicine or another field. It is time to embrace your uniqueness, harnessing its powers and capabilities to make your mark upon this world.

Kidney Transplant Breakthrough in 1954

Skin and eyes (cornea) were the first organs to be harvested and transplanted in the mid-1800s and early 1900s.[9] However, kidneys were the first large and more complex organ to be transplanted successfully.[9,10] Before the mid-twentieth century, if a patient had chronic kidney disease, there was little hope for a cure.[11] This changed with Dr. Joseph Murray in 1954.

Supported by the administration at Peter Bent Brigham Hospital and Harvard Medical School, Dr. Joseph Murray and a team of strategic surgeons successfully performed the first kidney transplant on identical twins, Richard and Ronald Herrick. Dr. Murray and his colleagues faced skepticism from the wider medical community in their attempt to remove a healthy kidney from a donor twin to benefit an unhealthy kidney recipient twin. Their doubts centered around the body's poorly understood rejection of foreign tissues, biological incompatibility, and immunological adaptability.[12]

Ultimately, Dr. Murray received the 1990 Nobel Prize in Physiology or Medicine. He paved the way for a new medical era.[11] Today, transplants are commonplace. There were 39,035 total transplants from January to December 2020 and 39,719 total transplants from January to December 2019.[13]

Lessons From Dr. Joseph Murray

Dr. Murray famously stated, "If you're going to worry about what people say, you're never going to make any progress."[11] Have you listened to the desires and goals of significant individuals in your life while suppressing your own? Have you asserted their wants and needs instead of your own? Have you absorbed each criticism, whether good or bad, with false gusto and drudgery? If the answer to any of these questions is yes, it is time to consider acting upon your wants and needs.

Helicobacter pylori Discovery and Breakthrough in 1982

Helicobacter pylori (H. pylori) is a gram-negative, curve-shaped bacterium usually colonized in the lower part of the human stomach.[14] It is an established cause of chronic active gastritis, chronic superficial gastritis, peptic ulcer disease, and gastric adenocarcinoma.[14,15] In fact, H. pylori causes approximately 90% of duodenal ulcers and more than 80% of gastric ulcers.[14] Although these diseases were prevalent in the 20th century, their medical history dates back to antiquity. One of the earliest descriptions of peptic ulcer disease was found in the 4th century BCE. It was carved on a pillar at the temple of Aesculapius, narrating the first gastric surgery. Another instance of peptic ulcer disease was found in the stomach of a mummy of the Western Han dynasty in 167 BCE.[14,15] The H. pylori link to stomach maladies remained elusive until Dr. Robin Warren and Professor Barry Marshall's discovery in 1982.[14,15]

Warren and Marshall conducted a study of 100 biopsies from patient stomachs comparing healthy and unhealthy guts. They observed a striking correlation: there was an increased presence of H. pylori from biopsies with gastritis. They discovered multiple signs of inflammation in the lower part of the stomach close to where they observed the bacteria.[16] Their research led to identifying a new bacterium.

The medical community was reluctant to receive Warren and Marshall's findings. They were unable to replicate their results in animal models. They received criticism and skepticism from scientific and clinical societies. Warren and Marshall's findings had attacked the medical world's entrenched belief that gastritis was mainly caused by lifestyle factors such as diet and stress.[14]

Consequently, Marshall took matters into his own hands and experimented on himself. In 1984, he initiated a series of baseline endoscopies showing a healthy gastric lining. Then, he drank a culture of the bacteria from an infected patient's biopsy. Within a couple of days, he developed nausea, vomiting, and easy fatigability — all symptoms of gastritis. A repeat endoscopy was performed and a biopsy taken. His results showed gastritis with positive H. pylori culture.[14,15,16] Marshall did not stop there. He began antibiotic treatment with bismuth and recovered completely.

Warren and Marshall's unorthodox, yet calculated, research greatly impacted the field of medicine.[16] In 1994, the National Institutes of Health officially recognized a causal link between H. pylori and ulcers. In 1996, the Food and Drug Administration approved an antibiotic therapy regimen to combat ulcers caused by H. pylori. In 2005, Marshall and Warren received the 2005 Nobel Prize in Physiology or Medicine.[14,16]

Lessons From Barry James Marshall and Robin Warren

Action drives results. Goals and passions must be coupled with action for an ultimate reaction. Consistent follow through with activity is essential. Development and growth will only be realized with continuous forward movement.

CHALLENGE 2:

Write down your core principles and values. Those values which are highly significant in your life will remain static no matter the changing circumstances. Writing down your static principles and values will ground you and equip you with the knowledge of things you cannot change, leaving room and innovation for the items you can.

CHALLENGE 3:

Write down the pros and cons of why you want an alternative career. Write your whys, so we can figure out your hows.

Chapter 2

Refocus Your Vision and Reinvent Your Perspective

The eagle has incredibly strong vision. Its visual acuity is four to five times greater than humans, giving it the ability to focus on an object five kilometers away. While the eagle sits high above a cliff, it sees everything below, around, and above it. Eagle eyes are designed for long distant focus and razor-sharp clarity. When the eagle spots prey from above, it narrows its focus quickly, holding it until he can grab the target, no matter the obstacle that hinders its way.[4] Eagles are miles ahead of their competitors in the animal kingdom. Are you ready to focus on your vision like the eagle?

A vision is a plan for your future with a set date as your goal. An effective vision is imaginable yet feasible, focused, and flexible. Begin by creating a hopeful picture of your future in your mind. Feel the interaction of sight, smell, taste, sound, and touch as you envision your dream becoming a reality. Is your vision attainable? Is it probable? Does it have a statistically significant chance of being achieved? Now, focus in on your vision with clarity, following it through to actions and interactions. See yourself making decisions and responding with reactions. Will your vision withstand the test of time? Can it survive challenges and obstacles?

The benefit of conceptualizing your vision is creating a tangible road map for decision-making. If I decide on this path, will it take me to my vision? If I decide on this detour, will my vision still be realized? Will this decision make a good or bad impact on my vision? Strategically mitigate risks through the conceptualization process. Is this risk worth taking? Is it worth foregoing? Your vision will become a guideline for your actions, interactions, and reactions. Maximizing your performance and creating partnerships that benefit your vision is your goal.

Why is this important? Because you want the best for your life. You do not want a superficial quick fix or a Band-Aid. You want a sustainable process that will optimize your outcome. You want a plan for the long term. You want a solution for a chronic condition.

A strong vision is needed to attain fulfillment in life and in your career. If you still do not know what you want to do, it is vital to understand what you want from work. For instance, what does your office space look like? Will you be working from home? Will you be working from a beach in Croatia or a cafe in Barbados? If it is in your current town, what is the environment of your new office? Is there a restaurant or a coffee shop nearby? Is your building lined with glass or wood? What is the size of the organization? What are your co-workers like? What types of people will you be working with? What kind of skills will you be using? Become the visionary of your own success.

When you say visionary, what traits come to mind? Focused. Risk-taker. Persistent. Bold. Strategic. Communicative. Organized. Collaborative. Innovative. Magnetic. Emotionally intelligent. Inspirational. Optimistic. Open-minded. When the word visionary is elicited, who comes to mind? Benjamin Franklin. Nikola Tesla. Martin Luther King. Winston Churchill. Steve Jobs. Bill Gates. Jeff Bezos. Elon Musk. Now let us consider three stories from the past, modern past, and present.

Benjamin Franklin (1706-1790)

Benjamin Franklin was one of the Founding Fathers of the United States of America. He was a political philosopher, a civic activist, a statesman, a governor, a diplomat, an ambassador, a scientist, an inventor, and a writer. He envisioned and avidly campaigned for America's colonial unity. Franklin was considered the "most influential in inventing the type of society America would become."[17]

Franklin was instrumental in building the foundations of colonial unity and defining the ethos of America. His visions for the emerging American nation were embodied in his diplomatic actions with France and Great Britain. He spearheaded the repeal of the Stamp Act from the Parliament of Great Britain. This was the taxation on documents for American commercial services.[18] His diplomacy was crucial in fostering the French-American relationship that was critical in securing munitions during the American Revolution.[17]

Lessons From Benjamin Franklin

If we asked Benjamin Franklin about visions, he would acknowledge, "By failing to prepare, you are preparing to fail."[19] You are now preparing for your vision to become your reality. When you put your heart, mind, and soul into achieving something, you are preparing yourself for success. When you create a strong vision, your thoughts, decisions, actions, and reactions will align to bring that vision to fruition.

Sir Winston Churchill (1874-1965)

Sir Winston Leonard Spencer-Churchill was a British military leader, statesman, and writer who served as Prime Minister of Great Britain twice – from 1940 until 1945 and again from 1951 until 1955. Churchill was instrumental in successfully leading Great Britain and Allied Forces to defeat Axis powers during World War II.[20]

Churchill's early story was not always one of success. He barely passed the admission examination for the Harrow Boarding school in 1888 and it took him three attempts to pass the admission exam for the Royal Military Academy in Sandhurst in 1893. He became a second lieutenant in World War I and served in Cuba, India, Egypt, and Sudan. He then served as a statesman for the House of Common, First Lord of Admiralty, Minister of Munitions, Chancellor of the Exchequer, and later, as Prime Minister.[20,21]

Churchill was an effective leader because he possessed strategic intuition. He vocally complained about the terms of the Munich Agreement, declaring that the agreement would not preserve Europe's uneasy peace while the threat of Nazi Germany was looming in the background. Moreover, during his "Iron Curtain" speech, he voiced his misgivings about Russia, which later proved correct during the Cold War.[20,21] Churchill's great foresight was a critical component of his leadership. His vision and refusal to surrender to Nazi Germany strengthened and inspired Great Britain. His insightfulness adequately prepared his country for war. He stated, "Adequate preparation for war is the only guarantee for preserving the State's wealth, natural resources, and territory."[20] In 1953, Churchill was named as the recipient of the Nobel Prize for Literature and was knighted by Queen Elizabeth II.[21]

Lessons From Sir Winston Churchill

Churchill coupled his foresight and vision with action and perseverance. He said, "You have only to endure to conquer. You have only to persevere to save yourselves and to save all those who rely upon you. You have only to go right on, and at the end of the road, be it short or long, victory and honor will be found."[22]

Elon Musk (1971-)

Elon Musk is a South African-born American immigrant, businessman, engineer, industrial designer, entrepreneur, and philanthropist. He pioneered several companies, including Zip2 in 1995, X.com in 1999, SpaceX in 2002, Tesla Motors in 2003, SolarCity in 2006, Open AI in 2015, and Boring Company in 2016. His company, X.com (which later became PayPal), revolutionized the global payment industry. His company, Tesla, is rapidly and strategically changing the face and performance of electric vehicles.[23]

According to Sir Richard Branson, "Whatever skeptics have said can't be done, Elon has gone out and made real. Remember in the 1990s, when we would call strangers and give them our credit card numbers? Elon dreamed up a little thing called PayPal. His Tesla Motors and SolarCity companies are making a clean, renewable-energy future a reality ... his SpaceX's reopening space for exploration ... it's a paradox that Elon is working to improve our planet at the same time he's building spacecraft to help us leave it."[23]

Lessons From Elon Musk

Musk's tactics to innovation and problem solving are a similar process to diagnosing a patient. A clinician defines the problem, completes a history and physical examination, orders laboratories and diagnostics to eliminate differentials, and provides evidence to the most likely cause of the disease. He then develops medical management suited for the individual patient. Musk defines a problem. He then learns, reads, and discovers everything surrounding the issue. He eliminates solutions by testing and retesting them in various situations. Finally, he comes up with the answer to manage said problem. The process of having an end goal keeps him focused and challenged.

Musk's visionary leadership has always challenged the status quo and embraced the need for change. He repeatedly tests and retests solutions to accelerate transformation. He is an avid champion of innovation through technology. But how? According to Jim Cantrell, "What I found from working with Elon is that he starts by defining a goal and he puts a lot of effort into understanding what that goal is and why it is a good and valid goal. Once he has a goal, his next step is to learn as much about the topic at hand as possible from as many sources as possible. He borrowed all of my college texts on rocket propulsion when we first started working together in 2001.... The one major important distinction that sets him apart is his inability to consider failure."[23]

CHALLENGE 4:

Write your vision statement. Finish this sentence:

In five years, I envision _____

In ten years, I envision _____

CHALLENGE 5:

Draw your vision.

Chapter 3

Redevelop a Growth Mindset and Restructure Your Neurons

The eagle embraces aging and change. When the eagle grows old, his worn and tempest-tossed feathers can no longer support his speed, altitude, and flight. The eagle retires to the highest cliff, plucks each old feather, and awaits new growth. When the new feathers grow, he soars to new adventures.[4] Like the eagle, are you ready to shed the old for the unknown? Are you prepared to develop a growth mindset and physically restructure your neurons?

Carol S. Dweck, PhD is a noted Stanford psychologist whose groundbreaking research looks at individual self-conception and its impact on achievement. A "growth mindset" is a term she coined that explains how we perceive ourselves. She argues that intelligence can be grown incrementally through positivity, training, and hard work. She contrasts this with a "fixed mindset" which assumes intelligence, creativity, and character are static and unchangeable. Dweck's work found that individuals with a fixed mindset tend to give up easily, avoid challenges, and have difficulty with constructive criticism, thereby falling short of their full potential. On the other hand, individuals with a growth mindset embrace challenges, persevere through hardship, and learn from criticism. As a result, they tend to achieve at higher levels. Growth-minded individuals perceive that challenges are part of the learning curve and vital to personal growth.[24]

Researchers have introduced the concept of neuroplasticity to induce a growth mindset. Neuroplasticity, also known as brain plasticity, is the brain's capability to change through restructuring and reorganizing of the brain's neural network. As we experience, learn, and adapt to new surroundings, our brain forms new connections. With neuroplasticity, each new thought and each new emotion creates a new neural pathway. The smallest change in how we perceive stimuli, if frequently repeated, can lead to permanent changes in how our brains work. It is like muscle building where repeated actions produce power and strength in the muscles.[25,26,27,28]

Teaching individuals the concept of neuroplasticity is a strategic tactic in developing a growth mindset. According to a meta-analysis study of ten peer-reviewed articles, inducing a growth mindset by teaching neuroplasticity has a comprehensive positive effect on motivation and achievement.[25] How we think about our brains affects how we learn. More simply, the more challenges we face, the stronger and smarter the brain becomes. As we continue to exercise our brains, new neural connections grow, and neuroplasticity occurs.

The growth mindset aims to replace the barriers of negative fixed thinking with a belief that you can grow. Dweck's body of work focuses on the power of one's beliefs and how profoundly they affect one's life. The process of going from a fixed mindset to a growth mindset will involve intentionally replacing negative thoughts with positive thoughts and focusing on your potential rather than where you are right now. It will involve the importance of risk, seeking out challenges, and the power of persistence. This self-insight will help you convert life's setbacks into future successes.[24,26]

Here are some examples of how you can leverage a growth mindset to restructure your neurons anatomically.

Intentional Thinking Through Mindful Meditation

Intentional thinking through mindful meditation is a mental practice of gaining influence over thoughts and emotions. You become aware of the thoughts that come to mind, you take responsibility for those thoughts, and you determine an action. Numerous studies show that long-term mindful meditation practice is correlated with altered electroencephalogram (EEG) trends, suggesting long-lasting changes in the brain's activity. A study by Garg in 2014 showed that individuals who meditate have improved signal transmission efficiency. Those who practice mindful meditation tend to experience decreased anxiety, improved emotional and behavioral balance, reduced insomnia, and reduced risk of depression.[29,30]

Another study by Sara Lazar et al. from Harvard University, in collaboration with the Dalai Lama, took 20 participants with extensive meditation experience and studied the effects of meditation on the brain.[31] Their brains underwent two MPRAGE (Magnetizations Prepared Rapid Gradient Echo) sequences. The resulting models were compared to an atlas of cortical folding patterns using a high-dimensional, non-linear registration technique. It elaborated on the link between meditation and the cortical thickness changes (or density) of the brain's gray matter. Gray matter is the portion of the brain that is composed of nerve cell bodies. The research showed that long-term meditation practice is important for sensory, cognitive, and emotional processing.[31]

Lessons About Intentional Thinking through Mindful Meditation

You have learned the importance of mindful meditation on neuroplasticity. Now, it is time to practice what you have learned.

1. Choose a comfortable environment where you will be uninterrupted. This should be a place where you feel peaceful and can detach from the hum of everyday occurrences. This could be a quiet part of your home or a bench in a park.

2. Choose a time. Set a meditation time of 10-15 minutes and work up from there. Choose small increments of time to commit to meditating. Schedule this meditation because what gets scheduled, gets done.

3. Choose a posture. There is no right or wrong meditation posture. Most associate meditating with a sitting lotus position where you sit with your legs crossed. Instead, do what feels natural and comfortable to you. Straighten your upper body. Relax your arms and legs. Play around with various postures.

4. Begin meditation. First, settle your mind. You may notice that detaching from a stressful day may take some time. Take this moment to identify your feelings and switch your attention to your physical position.

5. Focus on your breathing. Follow the path of your breath as you inhale and exhale. Feel the air as it comes in through your nose and fills your lungs. Inhale by counting to ten, hold your breath for ten seconds, then exhale by counting down from ten.

6. Take control of your thoughts and emotions. Appreciate your thoughts and feelings. There is no need to eliminate them. Let go of negative thoughts without judgment.

7. When a toxic thought enters your mind, you must first acknowledge it and then replace it with a healthy thought. Below are some examples of converting negative thoughts to positive thoughts.[27]

Fixed Mindset	Growth Mindset
My abilities, intelligence, and talents are fixed traits.	My abilities, intelligence, and talents can be developed through effort, learning, and persistence.
My potential is pre-determined.	My effort and attitude determine my potential.
Failure is the limit of my abilities.	Failure is an opportunity to grow.
When I am frustrated, I give up.	Challenges help me to grow.
I stick to what I know.	I like to try new things.
I am either good at it or I am not.	I can learn to do anything I want.

8. Focus on the present. Open your eyes, pausing to notice the sounds and the visions around you. Having centered and calmed your mind, go forth and continue your day.

Physical Activity

Aerobic exercise promotes neuroplasticity. A meta-analysis by Budde et al. examined six international pieces of research using different methods such as EEG readings, brain scans, and blood sampling and determined that physical exercise triggers neuroplasticity.[32] In another study, Erickson et al. found that physical exercise was a powerful process in increasing gray matter in the prefrontal cortex and hippocampus in individuals aged five to 80 years old. The same author completed meta-analyses of randomized controlled trials that concluded aerobic exercise interventions increase gray matter volume in adulthood and prevent brain atrophy.[33,34]

Another study by Lin et al. revealed physical exercise improved neuroplasticity in Alzheimer's patients by changing the synaptic structure, neurogenesis, and modulating glial activation that supports neuroplasticity. Firstly, it increased the production of neurotrophic factors such as vascular endothelial growth factor (VEGF), insulin-like growth factor 1 (IGF-1), and brain-derived neurotrophic factor (BDNF). Secondly, it changed cerebrovascular function and glial activation. Lastly, it decreased neuronal vulnerability by decreasing toxic proteolytic enzymes.[35]

Lessons About Physical Activity

The benefits of physical activity continue to grow. Make a conscious decision to exercise regularly. Again, schedule your exercise because what gets scheduled, gets done. Start with 10-15 minutes a day and build up to at least 30 minutes a day. Start by exploring a physical activity you enjoy such as walking, cycling, gardening, or swimming. Incorporate exercise into your daily routine. If you frequently work in front of a computer, take a 5-minute break once every hour. Sneak in a few exercises while cooking your food such as squats or lunges. Be creative with your physical activity. Keep your body moving.

Adequate Sleep

Sleep plays a critical role in brain growth and neuroplasticity. Chronic insomnia has been associated with neuronal damage and atrophy, while adequate quality sleep enhances neuroplasticity. A study by Guzman-Marin et al. determined that adult neuroplasticity was affected by sleep deprivation and sleep fragmentation. This study of sleep-deprived patients showed that proliferative and neurogenic processes were reduced by 50% and mature neuronal phenotypes were reduced by 35%.[36] Another study by Mueller et al. found that sleep deprivation was correlated with cognitive decline. They found strong evidence suggesting that sleep deprivation for more than 24 hours significantly blocked cell proliferation.[37]

Lessons About Sleep

Adequate sleep is a vital component of neuroplasticity. If you suffer from poor sleep, try going to sleep and getting up at the same time every day. This will reset your circadian rhythm and promote a healthy sleep-wake cycle. Avoid sleeping in on weekends and holidays. Try daytime naps rather than sleeping in to make up for a late night. Limit naps to 15-20 minutes in the early afternoon. Avoid bright screens, especially blue light emitted from laptops, phones, and TV within one hour of your sleep time. Keep your room at a comfortable temperature with adequate ventilation.[38]

CHALLENGE 6:

Whether on your phone or a planner, schedule two 10-15 minute meditation sessions and two 10-15 minute exercise sessions per week. Plan a specific time for bedtime and stick to it. Be consistent throughout the week. You've got this!

Chapter 4

Burnout Counselor

Overview

Job Title	Burnout Counselor
Salary Range	No literature found
Education	No requirements
Training	Those with experiences in counseling adapt easier to this role
Skills/Talents	Counseling, verbal and written communication, multi-tasking skills
Projected Job Growth	No literature found. See the Future Growth section for trends in the industry

What is a Burnout Counselor?

Let us first define burnout. Burnout is a state of physical, emotional, and mental exhaustion caused by excessive and prolonged stress. Burnout has detrimental effects on one's health, home, work, and social life.[39,40] In 2019, the World Health Organization included burnout in the International

Classification of Diseases as an occupational phenomenon.[41] When one is burned out, everything feels bleak and insurmountable. It is difficult to take action by oneself.

A burnout counselor is a professional who offers support and resources through a client's burnout process. They become a regular resource for encouragement and support to help clients regain contentment and fulfillment. The clientele for a burnout counselor can vary from junior doctors, general practitioners, specialists, trainees, consultants, and groups of physicians. It can also include clients in leadership roles like CEOs and other C-suite executives, supervisors, and managers. Burnout affects performance in and beyond the workplace and those struggling with it are willing to invest time to make their lives more manageable.

Sample Case

Amy Imms, MBBS earned her Bachelor of Medicine and Bachelor of Surgery degree with Honors from the University of Tasmania, Australia in 2007. She left her general practice (GP) training program after two years and became a burnout counselor. She said:

> I started following a traditional pathway. I was about two-thirds of the way through my general practice training program when I decided to stop and do something different. The things that led me to leave my GP training program were a combination of family, health issues, raising four young children, and trying to study for exams. I could not quite figure out how to fit everything in. I realized I was not enjoying what I was doing. I was not coping with life. I reassessed everything. I looked closely at work and what I enjoyed and did not like about it. What I found most fulfilling was this group of patients who had a similar experience to what I had experienced. They were struggling mentally, and they were burned out. It was hard for them to access resources to help them. I realized how hard it was finding good help in that situation. So I decided, I'm just going to go for it and see if I can make a career out of doing this one bit that I love. It was not a simple process. I went through a long period of questioning. If I leave, am I still a doctor? What are people going to think? Especially my family and my close friends, what are they going to think? So, it probably took me six months to make that decision and make that shift.[42]

Roles and Responsibilities

A burnout counselor offers one-on-one appointments, online programs, and group programs to guide clients through the journey from burnout to recovery. They also conduct workshops, teaching strategies to avoid burnout. They speak at conferences, businesses, and via podcasts about building healthy habits and coping skills to fight burnout. The burnout counselor explores a client's understanding of him/herself and assists him/her in realizing changes needed and in gaining perspective to allow that change to occur. They assist clients in reframing their perspectives and reevaluating their priorities. They help clients recognize the warning signs of burnout and formulate strategies for physical and emotional resilience.

Often, the burnout counseling session begins with the client telling their individual story. Dr. Amy was amazed to find that similar patterns emerged with her clients. She said:

> What are their challenges? How does their personality come into play? What aspects of their environment and their work are contributing to their situation? Usually, the types of things that end up coming up – particularly with doctors – are perfectionism, impostor syndrome, and setting boundaries. They either do not know their boundaries or they do not have the courage to maintain their boundaries. I focus on looking at what is in the workplace. It involves all of society. How have their past experiences shaped how they respond to events and what can they put in place to change that response? Some examples are mindfulness, going for a walk, or just doing something for fun. Several doctors have not enjoyed any of their hobbies or fun activities for a long time. We needed to re-introduce that.[42]

Skills, Education, Certification, and Training

There is no formal counseling qualification or training necessary to start as a burnout counselor. Burnout counseling is an independent business venture. Dr. Amy stated:

> I am not employed in my role. I run it all myself. So, in the beginning, I had to do everything. The biggest hardship was that everything fell on me. I was not sure how to go about starting this kind of business. Most advice I received from other people was completely different from medical practice guidelines. For example, things like laws regarding advertising and publishing testimonials, as well as how online businesses run and figuring out what I could do and what I could not do.[42]

The majority of the skills involved in becoming a burnout counselor are soft skills. The most obvious one is counseling skills. In fact, as healthcare professionals, we have experience counseling our patients. It is also equally important to exhibit compassion and care about people genuinely. The sessions are emotionally intense. Dr. Amy added:

> Another skill, just from the business side of things, is being decisive and able to make decisions. It is easy to get overwhelmed by different possibilities and avoid taking action. You must be able to act, plan ahead, and have a strategy for how your venture will work. There is no point in having a business that you love if it doesn't financially support you. You spend all this time, and you cannot pay your bills. So, you must have a clear plan and vision for how you are going to help people and make it viable business at the same time. Lastly, communication is key. You are constantly communicating with people, whether during talks or workshops or trying to build business relationships. This collaboration is a big part of burnout counseling. The relationships you build with other people are valuable.[42]

Pros and Cons

Some advantages to becoming a burnout counselor are:

1. The flexibility of time. With employment comes scheduled work hours from 9 a.m. to 5 p.m. with flexibility during lunchtime for personal errands. Do you remember squeezing in that dentist appointment by taking an early lunch? Having your own business and being your own boss provides you with a flexible schedule. You can customize your business plan to allow time for work, family, friends, and personal business. Your work schedule should work for your personal lifestyle and commitments.

2. Opportunity for remote work. Dr. Amy's burnout counseling business has been online since its inception five years ago utilizing telehealth. As a burnout counselor, you can work virtually as a digital nomad as long as you have a steady Wi-Fi connection.

Some challenges to becoming a burnout counselor are:

1. Burnout counseling is a new field with no guidelines. For some, the concept of exploring a new industry is exciting. For others, it is a daunting and overwhelming task. Perhaps the best part about the newness of burnout counseling is having the ability to define your own

path. You make the guidelines. You set your potentials and limits. You dictate your direction and process. Due to its newness, you will be spending a lot of time educating the public and creating awareness within your network and among prospective clients.

2. As aforementioned, burnout counseling is a business venture. You will need to learn how to multi-task. You must understand how to run a business through strategic marketing, financing, bookkeeping, and service development. You have a blank canvas in terms of how you choose to set up and run your practice.

Future Growth

Work-related burnout has increased at an alarming rate over the years. A 2020 survey by Gallup studied 7,500 full-time employees and found that approximately 66% dealt with burnout at some point at work.[43] Another 2020 study by Deloitte examined 1,000 full-time employees and found that 77% of the respondents experienced burnout, while 91% experienced unmanageable stress and frustration.[44] Interestingly, passion for one's work does not prevent workplace burnout. The same study by Deloitte showed that 87% stated they were passionate about their job, yet 64% stated they were frequently stressed.[44]

What about the clinical realm? At the beginning of 2020 (pre-COVID-19), Medscape surveyed 15,000 physicians from over 29 specialties. Their study showed that physician burnout had remained relatively consistent over the past five years at between 42-46%. Specifically, burnout statistics in the following specialties were higher than their counterparts: urology, neurology, critical care, internal medicine, family medicine, and emergency medicine.[45] Surprisingly, another study from Psychiatry Advisor stated that 40% of physicians are reluctant to seek mental health treatment for burnout because they harbor fears about job security and/or job loss.[46] With these numbers in mind, it can be concluded that this is a big issue presently and is only going to get worse. There is a real need for burnout counseling services.

Now What?

1. Decide if you have a passion for counseling. Counseling can be emotionally draining. You will be dealing with your clients' burnout stories. You will be sharing in their pains and discomforts. Is this something that you can comfortably commit to long term? Are you willing to listen to your client's despairs day in and day out with empathy, patience, and understanding?

2. Be open to feedback. If you are genuinely interested in exploring this option, ask your co-workers about your counseling skills. Take stock in whether you possess good counseling skills. If not, what can you do to become better at counseling?

3. Start your business, but do not quit your day job. The first months (often years) of starting your own business are financially challenging. To ease your transition, keep your day job to help pay for bills and necessities. Work outside of your regular work hours to grow your business. Dr. Amy advised:

   > Try not to doubt yourself too much. If you think this is what you want to do, then give it a go. If you have already got a medical registration or license, then I would always recommend trying to keep that going for at least a little bit so you have that option. If you decide this is not the profession for you, you will still have medicine to fall back on.[42]

4. Write a business plan. If you are unsure of how to go about starting this type of business, there are templates available online. The breadth and depth of writing a strategic business plan are beyond the scope of this book.

5. Connect with other business professionals in this industry. This chapter is an introduction to burnout counseling. Now, work and learn from the experts on how they started and what their initial and ongoing challenges have been. Inquire about their viewpoints on pricing and marketing strategies. If you wish to contact Dr. Amy, connect with me through my various social media platforms and I will bridge an introduction.

6. Rock it. Take the reins and gallop to reach the top. Show the world how amazing you are at this new venture. Make your mark in the burnout counseling industry.

About Dr. Amy

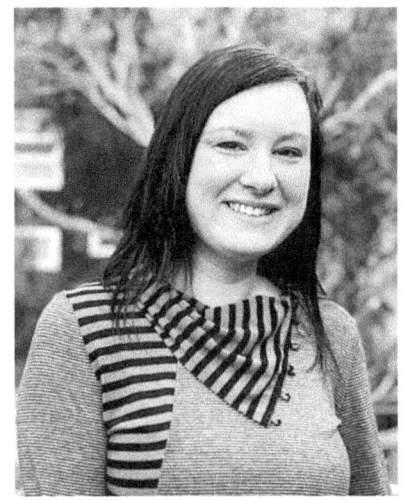

Amy Imms, MBBS earned her Bachelor of Medicine and Bachelor of Surgery degree with Honors from the University of Tasmania, Australia in 2007. She completed her internship and was a Resident Medical Officer for the Royal Hobart Hospital from 2008 to 2012. She trained as a general practitioner in Tasmania from 2013-2016. She started her burnout counseling business in 2016 and launched The Burnout Project in 2019. She is the author of *Burnout: Your First Ten Steps*. She has held a wide array of speaking engagements with the Rotary Club of Hobart (West Moonah Community House and Australian Rotary Health Wellness Expo), Creative Careers in Medicine Conference (Business over Breakfast, Grit and Growth Leadership Symposium, Tasmania Rural Health Conference), and media appearances with ABC local radio and the Sydney Morning Herald. Currently, she provides one-on-one and group burnout counseling programs all over Australia.

Dr. Amy also enjoys art, photography, running, and spending time in the beautiful Tasmanian bush and beaches. She homeschools her five children and is actively involved in the local home education community.

Chapter 5

Certified Life Coach and Cancer Coach

Overview

Job Title	Coach
Salary Range	Average annual income globally: $51,000[47]
Education/Training	Approximately 60 hours of education and ten hours of qualified mentor training through international coaching organizations. Upon completion, coaches will receive a certification[48,49]
Skills/Talents	Verbal communication, problem-solving, and analytical skills
Projected Growth	See the Future Growth section for trends in the industry

What are Certified Life Coaches and Cancer Coaches?

According to the International Coaching Federation, coaching is defined as a partnership between a coach and a client in a creative, yet thought-provoking, process to inspire and maximize a client's potential.[48] In the coaching continuum, some leaders and managers apply coaching skills to their workplace with varying training. For this chapter, coaches are classified as trained professionals who derive a portion of their annual income from internal or external coaching work.[49]

Coaching involves regular meetings between a client and a coach, designed to produce positive changes in a client's behavior within a limited time frame. The target audiences for coaches are managers

(29%), executives (23%), business owners/entrepreneurs (21%), and personal clients (19%). The majority of the clients (60%) are under 45 years old.[47] There is an average of 11 clients per coach at any given time.[50]

The coaching industry is becoming prevalent worldwide. The table below shows the estimates, by world region, of coach practitioners versus managers/leaders who utilize coaching skills.[48]

Coach practitioner and managers/leaders using coaching skills. Estimates by world region

	Coach practitioners	Managers/leaders using coaching skills	Coaching continuum
North America	17,500	3,100	20,600
Latin America and the Caribbean	4,000	1,000	5,000
Western Europe	18,800	2,700	21,400
Eastern Europe	4,500	1,500	6,000
Middle East and Africa	2,400	700	3,100
Asia	3,700	1,500	5,200
Oceania	2,400	400	2,800
Global	**53,300**	**10,900**	**64,100**

Note: Estimates are shown to the nearest 100. Therefore, subtotals may not add to the total figures.

There are three reasons why coaches are hired: to address a specific problem, to assist with a transition, or to attain a goal.[47] Coaching is a business venture. Other familiar sources of income for coaches include counseling, teaching, mentoring, training, facilitation, workshops, webinars, speaking engagements, and publications.

Coaching salaries vary by world region. The table below shows the average annual income (adjusted in US dollars) from the World Bank's exchange rates.[48]

Average annual revenue/income, USD Average

	USD
North America	$ 61,900
Latin America and the Caribbean	$ 27,100
Western Europe	$ 55,300
Eastern Europe	$ 18,400
Middle East and Africa	$ 35,900
Asia	$ 37,800
Oceania	$ 73,100
Global	**$ 51,000**

Coaching salaries vary widely depending on their specialty/niche. According to the Sherpa Executive Coaching Survey in 2018, an Executive Coach salary averaged $104,700, a Business Coach salary averaged $61,000, while a Life Coach salary averaged $37,000 USD.[47]

Sample Case

Anitha R, MBBS earned her Bachelor of Medicine and Bachelor of Surgery degree and her Master of Surgery (Otorhinolaryngology) degree from the Maharaja Sayajirao University of Baroda in Gujarat, India but pivoted to become a Certified Life Coach and Cancer Coach. Dr. Anitha stated:

> It occurred to me that medicine is great. We are made to diagnose a disease and manage it. But I always felt that there was something more. Why is the person even developing that disease? And back then, the mind-body connection was not part of the differential diagnosis. It was never part of our curriculum. I felt I was incomplete. Even though I was treating patients, I felt like there was so much more that I could do.[51]

Dr. Anitha started her self-search. She underwent coaching during her own battle with cancer and found the process fascinating. She began attending several workshops in coaching and the pieces of her future began to come together. She stated:

> I retained my full-time position as a surgeon. I took my coaching classes on weekday evenings. If my internet acted up, I would go to a coffee shop. But I never missed a single class. I just absolutely loved it.[51]

Roles and Responsibilities

The coaching process starts with the first (often complimentary) 20–30-minute consultation. The first session's goal is to determine if there is a match between the coach and the client. Dr. Anitha stated:

> As a life coach, I need to make clear with the client what they are looking for. Coaching is not therapy. Coaching is not counseling. It is also important to know how coachable the client is and how much commitment he/she can apply. How much is the client willing to invest? It is about getting a clearer idea of what I am signing up for and what the client is signing up for. We

determine whether we are a good fit and whether the client wishes to meet one-on-one or in a group. Working in a group can have beautiful dynamics when clients are going through the same journey. With one-on-one, clients have the full attention of the coach. It's a tailor-made session. Some people feel three or four sessions will be good enough. Some people feel we need to be together for at least six months. We talk about how often we need to meet. And then from there, I know where they want to be headed. They know what they are signing up for and I know what to look forward to and how to prepare as well.

We all have our goals. As a life coach, I am not trying to teach you. I'm not saying that you should be doing this, or you shouldn't be doing that. I am just trying to get it out of you. Coaching asks what is it that you want? How do you think you can go about getting it? What support do you need? What support can I give you? [51]

Dr. Anitha explained that she helps the client manifest becoming one with themselves. She serves as a stability and accountability partner for the client, while being her own boss with her own voice. As a cancer coach, Dr. Anitha said:

My main goal is relaying to my client that I may be a doctor, I may be a surgeon, but I am not here to give medical advice. Part of this statement is on my agreement as well. Cancer is a part of a cancer client's every living moment, every day. The only time they may not be thinking about it is when they sleep. An important step for a client is accepting and affirming the presence of cancer. You would not envision that diagnosis on your worst enemy, but having accepted the diagnosis, is the client willing to continue being in that space of fear? Or is he/she willing to convert it and face this challenge in life? What are the tools that the client wants to capitalize on? What do they think is going to help them through their cancer journey?

I help women and men who were previously healthy only to be struck by cancer. I help them by using anchors like their dream vacations and nature to connect them to a safe place where healing can happen. I help them, in a very loving way, deal with identity shifts that happen automatically with a cancer diagnosis. I help them practice gratitude and always lead them to an optimistic point of view. I help them see that they can still dream.

The most crucial thing is the fact that they feel listened to, they feel heard, and they know they will emerge learning something in the end. They know what they share is confidential. They know that they are not being judged. They can say what they want. They can swear. They can cry. They can shout. They can do whatever they want and it is all okay. I make sure that at the end of it all, they feel good. They feel that they have been listened to. They can make friends with faith and hope. All this helps them ease the journey.[51]

Skills, Education, Certification, and Training

There is no mandatory training or certification to become a Life Coach or a Cancer Coach. However, to increase your credibility and reputation with your clients, international organizations offer certifications. Accordingly, 77% of coach practitioners responded that clients expect them to be credentialed or certified. Approximately 89% of all coach practitioners received accredited or approved training from a professional coaching organization. The survey also showed that consumers are more than likely to recommend a credentialed coach versus a non-credentialed coach.[49]

Some of the more reputable international organizations include the International Coaching Federation (ICF) and the International Association of Coaching (IAC). ICF is a global non-profit organization dedicated to building a worldwide network of trained coaching professionals. They provide independent certification to professional coaches and accreditation to coach training programs.[48] As of July 2020, there were 41,500 members from 147 countries. ICF has three credentialing programs: Associate Certified Coaches (ACC), Professional Certified Coaches (PCC), and Master Certified Coaches (MCC).[49] The hours of education and training vary by credentialing programs. After completing the agenda, the prospective coaches take a 155-multiple choice, web-based examination to complete the certification process.[48]

IAC is a global coaching association that provides certification and membership to a coach's ongoing pursuit of mastery. IAC gives credit for prior coaching training and emphasizes mastery over documentation. They also aim to build a diverse global network of professional coaches. As of November 2020, IAC membership totaled 25,855 coaches in over 80 countries.[52]

There are other global organizations within niche markets including the Association of Coach Training Organizations (ACTO), Health Coach Alliance (HCA), The European Mentoring and Coaching Council United Kingdom, The Gay Coaches Alliance, and the Professional Association of ADHD Coaches (PAAC).[48]

Pros and Cons

Some advantages to becoming a coach are:

1. Flexibility of time. With this career, you choose when to work. You can work three to four times a week with two to three clients a day. Or you can work two to three times a week with three to four clients a day. You dictate your schedule and your sessions.

2. Flexibility of setting. Coaches can use a virtual platform to meet with clients across the globe. Or you can opt to see clients face-to-face, so as not to lose the human connection. You can conduct one-on-one sessions or group sessions.

3. There is a constant integration of health skills and coaching methodology. Although you are not working as a clinician, your clinical knowledge, background, and experience will lend unique insight to the coaching profession.

Some challenges to becoming a coach are:

1. Coaching is an independent business venture. You will need to learn how to run your own coaching business, including marketing, bookkeeping, accounting, publicity, and service development. You need to multi-task, from creating a website to booking clients to developing a referral system. This can be a tremendous learning experience which allows your creativity and innovation to be unleashed. Your strategies and ideas will be awakened. The possibilities are endless.

2. Most coaches work independently. This may be advantageous for some, but for a newbie in the coaching profession this can be a daunting task to undertake. However, with professional certification and mentor training you will feel more confident with your first client.

Future Growth

The coaching industry is growing at an exponential rate. The business coaching market was worth $15 billion in 2019.[50] However, with the global e-learning market – a combination of online coaching and digital learning platforms – it is estimated to reach more than $325 billion by 2025.[53] There is increased global awareness of the benefits of coaching. There is also credible data on the return of investment from working with a professional coach. This improved market perception and positive media has increased demand for coach practitioners.[47,50]

Expected future trends for 2022 and beyond include an estimated increase of 82% in professional coaching for millennial leaders and 83% for team coaching. We will also see an increase of 89% in the prevalence of all coaching programs.[49]

Now What?

1. Reflect and ask yourself these questions: Am I passionate about helping clients pursue and manifest their solutions? Am I driven to help clients work through problems to attain their fullest potential? Am I able to help clients put their pieces together and transition them to a fulfilling life? Do I have the knowledge and skills to start a coaching business?

2. Join an international coaching organization. Whether it is ICF or IAC, join a globally recognized professional platform to connect with other coaches. The organization will provide resources and tools for guidance and support throughout your coaching journey.

3. Earn the credentials needed and the training required to become a certified coaching professional. Take the 60-hour educational coursework and the ten-hour mentor training from an international coaching organization. This involvement will arm you with the knowledge and experience to be confident with your first client. Certification will lend you credibility in the industry.

4. Explore your niche. Find your passion for a specific market. Be boldly unique and different. Be ready to be a subject-matter expert in your prospective niche. Some examples of niches include cancer coaching, health and wellness coaching, and weight loss coaching.

5. Network. Building strong connections and partnerships within your community will transition you to a successful coaching career. Approximately 80% of coaches gain clients through personal referrals.[50]

6. Strategically market and publicize your services. To get a little, sometimes you have to give a lot. Utilize social media platforms to create content about coaching. Write articles on self-identity and self-empowerment. Write articles on topics you can confidently speak about. When clients consume your content, they will gravitate to you to learn more about you and your services. Respond and share articles from other coaches. This will boost your social media presence and may land you a referral or two.

7. Enjoy the journey. Learn from your setbacks and challenges. When you fall, get back up and try again and again. Concentrate on your strengths and work to improve your weaknesses. Be the best version of yourself and don't be afraid to show the world how amazing you are.

About Dr. Anitha R

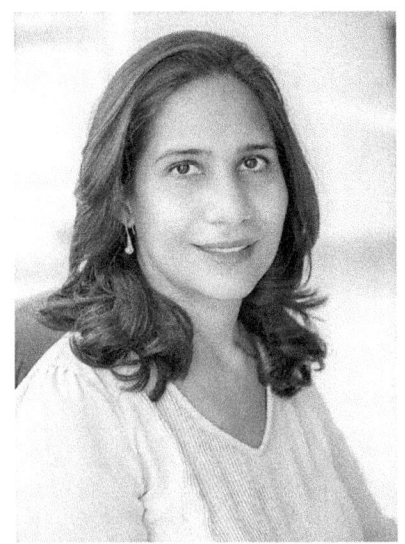

Dr. Anitha R is co-author of *The Shakti Awakening*, an international #1 best seller on Amazon in several categories. She is an ICF Certified Life Coach from Symbiosis Coaching and has undergone extensive mentor training as a Cancer Coach. She has seen cancer in different ways – she has diagnosed cancer, conducted surgeries on cancer, and survived cancer herself.

Anitha R, MBBS earned her Bachelor of Medicine and Bachelor of Surgery degree and her Master in Surgery degree in Otorhinolaryngology from the Maharaja Sayajirao University of Baroda in Gujarat, India. She also received her Diplomate of the National Board (Otorhinolaryngology) in 1999. Her career in medicine spans almost 20 years in numerous hospitals and reputable medical universities in Malaysia and India. She has been an invited speaker at various conferences and has been featured in multiple podcasts.

Dr. Anitha has been actively involved in research and her work is published in peer-reviewed journals. She moved to New Zealand in 2017 and worked as Director of the Advanced Clinical Skills Centre at the University of Auckland until 2019. Throughout her career, she actively volunteered in many international medical camps. She is very passionate about making a difference.

Dr. Anitha is multilingual and speaks five languages. She spends her leisure time with her family and considers herself a lifetime learner who enjoys solitude, kundalini yoga, baking, and forest walks. Having been diagnosed with cancer in February 2020, Dr. Anitha is passionate about helping and empowering those whose bodies have been afflicted with this disease. She believes that cancer is not a death sentence and that if she can beat cancer anybody can.

CHAPTER 6

Clinical Content Manager

Overview

Job Title	Clinical Content Manager / Medical Content Manager / Clinical Content Specialist / Healthcare Content Manager
Salary Range	Average annual income in the US: $56,779. Ranges from $38,000 (10th percentile) to $84,000 (90th percentile)[54]
Education	MD/DO required. Clinical experience is a bonus
Training	On-the-job training available in some companies, while most companies require 1-2 years of content management experience
Skills/Talents	Writing skills, analytical skills, attention to detail, creativity, organizational skills, research skills
Sample Companies	Athena health, Change Healthcare, Concentra, Cotiviti, Docquity, Elsevier, Kaiser Permanente, McKesson, M*Modal, Performance Health, Truven Health Analytics, WebMD, Wolters Kluwer
Projected Job Growth	No literature found. See the Future Growth section for trends in the industry

What is a Clinical Content Manager?

A clinical content manager oversees the production of high-quality, evidence-based content for target audiences. They are advocates of medical journalism who are passionate about communicating clinical ideas and updated information to globally shape health and health care. Clinical content managers often work for pharmaceutical, insurance, research, medical device/medical education companies, and healthcare delivery organizations. They also partner with reputable and specialty associations. Their purpose is to teach, educate, and share clinical knowledge with the general public.

Sample Case

Dr. Patrick Indradjaja earned his Doctor of Medicine degree from Trisakti University in Jakarta, Indonesia. He transitioned from medicine to research, and then medical content management. He stated:

> I fell in love with research. I earned my master's degree in research from Newcastle University in the United Kingdom. I was interested in stem cell research for disease modeling and future therapies. I became a researcher for three years. Researchers in my country, Indonesia, are not well paid so I changed to my current career working in the healthcare tech industry.[55]

Dr. Patrick was looking for an alternative career that would offer more financial stability and sustainability. He was introduced to his current healthcare organization by a friend's sister. Dr. Patrick stated that he started as head of content management. He managed all content for mobile and website platforms, edited content from his team, and scheduled content flow.[55]

Roles and Responsibilities

A clinical content manager's world revolves around medical journalism from inception to implementation and monitoring. Their responsibility falls under five categories: researching, editing, optimizing, writing, and updating. The content manager primarily utilizes his/her research skills and creativity to identify critical health topics to write about. They research scholarly resources and journals to provide in-depth evidence and knowledge about medical and health issues. They read and critically appraise peer-reviewed articles.[56] Dr. Patrick reported that clinical content managers research, find good journals, and critically review the journals.[55]

Secondly, they review, assess, and appraise their team's articles for accuracy, quality, completeness, and timeliness. This editing requires clinical intuition to understand when something is off. They also make sure all content is cited accurately. Thirdly, they strategically present information by optimizing content organization, structure, and reading level. They understand the power of diagrams, charts, images, and other visual media to boost the article's reception.[56]

Moreover, clinical content managers write articles. Although they write less than medical writers, they may still communicate complex medical and scientific information to the general public. They develop, implement, and monitor new content. Lastly, they update, repurpose, and clean up outdated content, making sure content remains relevant with updated facts and figures.[56]

Dr. Patrick went on to say that he also communicates with different associations and societies. He plans events, webinars, and conferences. He works with industry experts to provide audiovisual content and schedules video recording sessions for events and webinars.[55]

Skills, Education, Certification, and Training

Most job openings seeking a clinical content manager require an MD/DO degree with clinical experience. There is no formal training or certification required for this career. Most companies also require 1-2 years of content management experience – whether writing, researching, or editing medical content. It is imperative to have excellent writing and editing skills to succeed in this career. The ability to organize and strategically structure the content for optimal engagement is a plus. Understanding your target audience to align with their drives, likes, and dislikes is imperative in gaining optimal attention.

Pros and Cons

Some advantages to becoming a clinical content manager are:

1. Remote work. Most clinical content management can be done remotely, as long as you have a laptop and Wi-Fi access. Some organizations require office presence for meetings and events, but more and more are transitioning to remote work. This requires effective independent time management to reach the desired quantity and quality of articles produced.

2. Your research experience will come in handy. Most organizations are looking for individuals with writing and research skills. You can leverage your research skills with assessments and appraisals of peer-reviewed journals. Your other research skills, including data collection, data interpretation, literature reviews, and analysis will be transferrable to this career.

3. Your clinical knowledge will come in handy. Since this career communicates medical knowledge and information, you will be an asset because you will not have to fact-check every piece of information (unless you are unsure of its accuracy). If you have worked in clinics, you may determine what the public is looking for in clinical content.

Some challenges to becoming a clinical content manager are:

1. Be prepared to read a lot. This may be a pro for some individuals who love to read and learn, but the amount of medical content you need to ingest and digest is massive. Daily, you read articles from various reputable resources to gauge industry needs and wants. On average, you will need to read five to ten articles to comprehensively write and produce a single piece of content.

2. Be prepared to meet deadlines for your outputs. Dr. Patrick explained that you must create content daily. You also must read a lot of information and summarize material in terms everyone can understand.

Future Growth

Massive digital information consumption has increased the demand for health and healthcare content. Approximately 93 million Americans search for health-related topics online each year.[57] Consumers expect immediate responses to their healthcare questions. The most accessed resource tool searches for health-related content are WebMD (56%), Wikipedia (31%), web-based health magazines (29%), Facebook (17%), and YouTube (15%).[58]

Although consumers are hungry for health-related content, supply is not keeping up with demand. The Content Strategist Report by Contently analyzed 1,551 healthcare contents from 15 healthcare companies. Data showed that 63% of healthcare companies listed on the Fortune 1000 list had no owned content on their website or had limited content presence.[59] With this in mind, there is an apparent gap between demand and supply for health and healthcare-related content. There is tremendous opportunity in this industry mainly because patients need accurate and proactive information on health-related topics.

Now What?

1. Compile your medical writing portfolio. Whether it's a clinical case study in medical school or research work during post-graduate training, collect your medical writing projects. This will come in handy when you are applying for jobs, as employers will want to see examples of your medical journalism prowess.

2. Instead of researching positions on LinkedIn or Indeed.com, try researching organizations and going through their careers page on their individual websites. Some organizations do not readily post their openings on job boards.

3. Find recruiters through LinkedIn and request a "connection." Look for recruiters with experience working with start-up companies. Add a personal touch by researching them thoroughly before making contact. Ask them questions about what they do and how they are involved with their community.

4. Network with someone from your prospective organization. The best resource is LinkedIn. Search for the company name in the search bar, and filter using the "People" icon. This will give you a comprehensive list of possible connections. Send a "Connect" invite and always "Add a Note." The "Add a Note" section is a free tool on LinkedIn. Write a short paragraph on why you are reaching out. Here is an example:

   > Hello Sir/Madam,
   >
   > I am looking to expand my connections in the field of medical journalism. I saw that you work for XYZ organization. I would love to connect, hear about your experiences, and gain advice on how to leverage my medical degree for this career. Can we do a virtual coffee?
   >
   > Sincerely,
   > Your name

   Your goal is to give your time to get their time. Set up a Zoom virtual coffee. Listen to their story. Then, share your story and what you are looking for. Genuinely get to know the person. Keep in touch with them every month. You will create a lasting impression and be first on their call list when there are future openings within their organization.

About Dr. Patrick

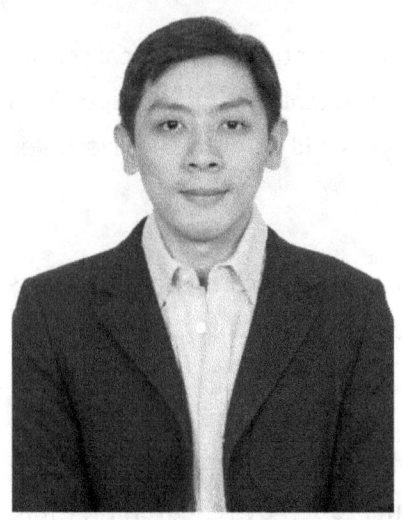

Patrick Indradjaja, MD, MRes earned his Doctor of Medicine degree from Trisakti University in Jakarta, Indonesia. He also holds a Master of Research in Stem Cell Biology and Regenerative Medicine degree from Newcastle University in the United Kingdom. He completed his internship in Clinical Pathology from Rumah Sakit Cipto Mangunkusumo Hospital (2010-2011). He worked as a general practitioner for the Departemen Kesehatan (2011-2012), Borromeus Hospital (2012-2014), and Rumah Sakit Cahya Kawaluyan (2013-2014). He also volunteered as a general practitioner for Tim Bantuan Medis Trisakti Hospital.

Dr. Patrick transitioned from medicine to become Head of Content in Docquity. Currently, he is Head of Partnership Content and Creative Development for Docquity.

In his free time, he takes courses to become a cardiac Pilates instructor. His hobbies include plant collecting and selling and he dreams of owning his own nursery one day.

Chapter 7

Entrepreneur

Overview

Job Title	Entrepreneur
Salary Range	Varies by industry, location, experience, and success of the business
Education / Training	Varies by industry
Skills/Talents	Project management, verbal and written communication skills, analytical and multitasking skills, perseverance, and insightfulness
Projected Job Growth	See the Future Growth section for trends in the industry

What is an Entrepreneur?

An entrepreneur starts or operates a business while bearing most of the financial and personal risks and enjoying most of the rewards. Entrepreneurs are innovative business people with fresh new ideas, products, and procedures. They are brilliant individuals who accomplish extraordinary things because they are passionate about what they do. Entrepreneurs are also risk-taking optimists who commit to working long hours to reach their desired outcomes. They combine capital and labor to produce goods and services for the purpose of making a profit.[60]

Sample Case

Dr. Vu Tran is co-founder, Director, and Chief Growth Officer for Go1 Pty. Ltd. Go1, founded in 2009, is the world's largest marketplace of workplace learning, servicing over 2 million people globally with offices in Australia, United States, Europe, Africa, and Southeast Asia.[61] He earned his Bachelor of Medicine and Bachelor of Surgery (MBBS) degree from Bond University, Australia in 2011 and attained his Fellow of the Royal Australian College of General Practitioners in 2016. He still practices medicine part-time as a general practitioner with Chatswood Road Medical Centre in Queensland, Australia. According to Dr. Vu:

> I have never not practiced medicine since I graduated medical school. I have never taken time off. I have never stopped. I have just reduced the frequency through which I practice. I am very proud of what we are building at Go1 and what we are doing as a company, but I'm also very thankful for the opportunity to switch gears once a week and focus on being a doctor and helping people. I love that because it is my one opportunity each week where I do not think about my company. Medicine is a form of mindfulness.[61]

When asked how he started his business, Dr. Vu stated:

> I run this business with my best friends from high school. We started our first business before I started medical school when I was 17. We have always wanted to work in technology and build a business, so when it comes to how we got to where we are, for me it was sheer dumb luck in terms of the people who have gravitated towards us. But it has not been without a lot of hard work and effort balancing medical school and growing a business. Now, we are the world's largest training provider of workplace training as a marketplace. Think of us as Netflix or Spotify for workplace learning. We bring over a hundred thousand different courses in learning items to employees in workplaces across the world.[61]

Roles and Responsibilities

In American society, entrepreneurship has been dramatically romanticized with companies like Google and Facebook which made their founders very wealthy. Unlike traditional careers and professions where you have a defined path to follow, the road to successful entrepreneurship is bumpy, often treacherous, and filled with roadblocks and dead ends.[60]

Ultimately, entrepreneurship is significantly individualized – what works for one person may not work for another. Here are some examples of the roles and responsibilities of an entrepreneur:

1. An entrepreneur needs financial stability. He/she must have adequate cash flow and capital to build a business, providing a cushion for start-up costs and time to work on innovation. There is no such thing as quick money. There are several ways to gain financial stability, such as pitching ideas to potential investors, crowdfunding, and small business loans. As the business progresses, it is important to be shrewd about money management. Keep social and business costs separate. Maintain rigorous bookkeeping practices and follow a strict operating budget.[60]

2. Entrepreneurs diversify their skill sets. They are both the boss and the worker. They are the Chief Executive Officer, webmaster, accountant, salesperson, and marketing representative. They are the brain and the brawn of the company. Outsourcing to external talent comes later as the entrepreneur engages more customers and consumers.

3. Entrepreneurs are consumers of content. They need to understand their target audience and their industry. Through podcasts, articles, books, lectures, and webinars, entrepreneurs gain valuable knowledge about the world around them for a fresh perspective. They are content experts whose goal is to influence the thoughts, behaviors, and actions of their target audience to use their products and services.[60]

4. Entrepreneurs identify problems quickly. They utilize their knowledge and experience in the industry to resolve specific problems as they arise. They build a business around solving an industry pain point for other businesses and consumers. They find solutions and make them available for general consumption.[60,62]

Skills, Education, Certification, and Training

There is no formal education, certification, or training to become an entrepreneur. However, an entrepreneur must possess passion for his/her chosen field to fuel internal drives into action. Passion provides the superior energy and stamina that overcomes challenges and continuously strengthens the entrepreneur's pursuit of goals. Passion gets the individual going even when income is slow or the business is losing money. There are no employer-sponsored benefits to fall back on. Entrepreneurs work tirelessly to achieve their purpose. Dr. Vu stated:

> You must have a clear sense of purpose in whatever you are doing. I wanted to practice medicine because I wanted to make a difference. My worlds come together by taking that sense of being able to make a difference as a doctor and then having the opportunity to do that on a bigger scale with my company. If I see 30 patients a day as a general practitioner and multiply that by 300 days a year, I might help the lives of 9,000 people. How do I potentially change the lives of 900 million people? That is genuinely our goal as a company: to help train a billion people globally.[61]

One of the biggest challenges of building a new business is sustaining the momentum and passion for innovation. Dr. Vu went on to say:

> I see everything I do as a marathon, not a sprint. For me, the biggest challenge is finding time to have the cognitive load left to be able to deal with whatever problem I am dealing with as a doctor and the load to be able to deal with running a business. But one caveat is that I have three fellow co-founders who are able to share the workload. I am privileged to have awesome co-founders and brilliant people to lean on.[61]

Pros and Cons

Some advantages of becoming an entrepreneur are:

1. Be your own boss. An entrepreneur is someone who consciously chooses freedom. Most people spend years building other people's dreams and following someone else's rules. Entrepreneurs choose to live their dream in their way. They set their own goals, control their progress, and run their business as they deem fit. They also understand that their business' success or failure is dependent upon their actions.

2. Flexible hours and location. Entrepreneurship allows individuals to work when they can, while juggling demanding schedules and responsibilities. It is also popular with individuals who do not want to be tied down to one place or location. It provides flexibility to be anywhere at any time you choose.

3. Step in and out anytime. If you have steady employment with a guaranteed salary, entrepreneurship is a career whereby you can pursue something new. You have a stable and secure path to fall back on while exploring your creativity and innovation.

Good doctors make good salespeople. According to Dr. Vu:

> The term 'bedside manner' focuses on communication skills. Universities are making sure they produce doctors who are good communicators. The interview process to get invited to any program is the medical school's way of understanding whether you're capable enough to communicate to patients and effectively convey a message so that they will buy into your advice. One of the best things I can do for a patient who comes in with a cold and wants antibiotics is to explain that antibiotics will do nothing for their cold. The best sale I can make is to convince a patient to understand that antibiotics do not kill viruses. They need to look after themselves and manage themselves symptomatically. That is a sale for me.[61]

4. Create a legacy. Whether through gaining financial stability and security for your heirs, creating a brand that will outlast a lifetime, or leaving behind innovation that improves lives, entrepreneurs make something with a lasting impression.[62]

Some challenges of becoming an entrepreneur are:

1. Starting a new business and keeping it going are the two biggest challenges. There is no such thing as overnight millionaires in entrepreneurship. There are a lot of sleepless nights and plans that do not work out. Building a business takes time, effort, perseverance, sacrifice, and good business acumen.

Future Growth

There were 582 million entrepreneurs in the world in 2020. Furthermore, 67.7% of the world's wealthiest individuals (worth at least $30 million USD) are self-made entrepreneurs. More than half of the new businesses started in the United States over the past decade are owned by African Americans, Latin Americans, and Asian Americans.[63] With these statistics in mind, there is enough room for your business and your entrepreneurial mindset.

Now What?

1. Name your business.

    a. Choose a business name that accurately represents your products and services, yet is memorable enough to stand out to customers.

    b. Make sure no other business in your location has the same name. This may involve searching through federal and state business databases.

    c. Join social media platforms by opening accounts under your business name. Social media platforms such as Facebook, Instagram, Twitter, and LinkedIn are possible marketing platforms to build your presence and brand.

    d. Secure a domain name and email address. As a new business, you want to build a website to establish your online presence and give your customers a look and feel to your business. If you opt not to have a website, it is still advisable to purchase a domain name so that no one else can have that business presence. You can search and register for a domain name through Google Domains, Web.com, or Godaddy.com.

2. Write a business plan. A business plan is a written document that states a business' objectives and goals. It should be a detailed plan with an executive summary, market analysis, detailed descriptions of products and services, marketing strategies, financial planning, and a budget.[64] You can search Google.com or Etsy.com for business plan templates.

3. Company formation.

    a. Incorporate your business. Apply to incorporate your business, whether as a Limited Liability Company (LLC), a corporation, or a nonprofit. Some websites allow you to apply for this, such as Incfile.com and Legalzoom.com.

    b. Obtain a Federal Employer Identification Number (EIN)/Tax ID Number. Whether you decide to hire employers later or not, this number allows you to identify your business as an entity for tax purposes.

c. Satisfy all business licensing and permitting requirements by state or region. You will need to call the Small Business Administration in your state or region to find out the requirements, licenses, and permits to run your business.

d. Establish a company address or virtual mailbox. Some companies offer virtual mailboxes – they scan your mail and send them to you by email, depending on your subscription.

4. Financials.

    a. Open a business bank account. Having a separate business account from your personal account will make matters more manageable when it comes to filing tax returns. This will isolate accounting, invoices, and sales, integrating them into one specific account for reporting purposes.

    b. Secure a business loan or other funding. You can apply for a small business loan, a traditional loan, or qualify for a line of credit. You can also raise capital through investors or angel investing or borrow from people you know.

    c. Learn bookkeeping. You can opt to sign up for accounting and invoicing software or do your bookkeeping on your own through Excel. The critical part of bookkeeping is keeping track of your spending and sales.

5. Operations. Find office space, purchase equipment, and find the best business software. The operational aspect of your business depends on what kind of business you want to run.

6. Marketing.

    a. Design a business logo. Your logo is the first part of your branding, so it is vital to invest in this process. You can find a graphic designer through Fiverr.com or Upwork.com.

    b. Build a company website. As mentioned before, you need an online presence to build your business. Aside from making social media handles, build a comprehensive, user-friendly website.

7. **Have a can-do attitude.** Dr. Vu stated:

> Doctors, in general, are quite smart people. Therefore, the likelihood of you making a stupid decision is quite low. One of the key reasons you might not be successful is not committing enough or not putting in the right amount of energy, effort, and time. Trust your gut in making the right decisions. Your instincts as a doctor have gotten you to where you are today. The law of probability is that you are going to make the right decisions because you are a good decision maker. I'm saying you need to explore.[61]

About Dr. Vu

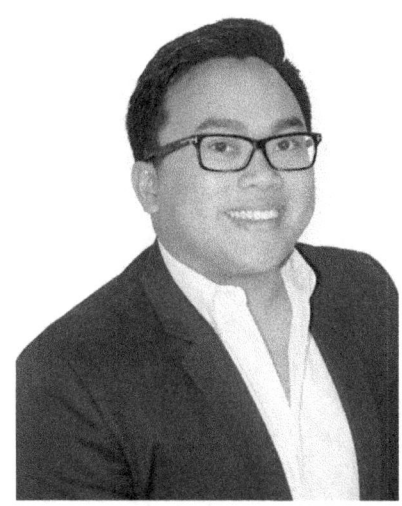

Vu Tran, MD, FRACGP is co-founder, Director, and Chief Growth Officer of Go1, the world's largest provider of workplace training, servicing over 2 million people globally with offices in Australia, United States, Europe, Africa, and Southeast Asia. In 2019, Go1 became the first Australian company to receive investment from Microsoft (M12) and is recognized by LinkedIn as one of Australia's top start-ups (2018 and 2019).

Dr. Vu was awarded the Brisbane Young Entrepreneur of the Year Award in 2019 and was a finalist every year from 2009-2019. He also received the Queensland Vietnamese Community Award for Academic Achievement in 2007.

Dr. Vu has practiced medicine part-time as a general practitioner for Chatswood Road Medical Centre in Queensland, Australia from 2015 to the present, Alderley Clinic in 2015, and Queensland Health from 2012-2014. He earned his MBBS (Bachelor of Medicine and Bachelor of Surgery) degree from Bond University, Australia in 2011 and attained his Fellow of the Royal Australian College of General Practitioners in 2016.

Chapter 8

Global Health Advisor

Overview

Job Title	Global Health Advisor / Public Health Advisor / Global Health Consultant / Public Health Consultant
Salary Range	Annual average income in the US: $79,993. Ranges from $49,500 (25th percentile) to $146,000 (90th percentile)[65]
Education	Most require an advanced degree, Master of Public Health (MPH)
Training	Most require global health experience
Skills/Talents	Program management skills, verbal and written communication skills, problem-solving and critical thinking skills, cultural intelligence
Sample companies	American Red Cross, Africare, Bill and Melinda Gates Foundation, Bread for the World, CARE, Center for Disease Control and Prevention (CDC), Christian Children's Fund (CCF), Family Health International, Global Health Council, Mercy Corps, National Institute of Health (NIH), Oxfam, PATH, Project HOPE, Save the Children, Partners in Health (PIH), US Agency for International Development (USAID), US Department of Health and Human Services, World Bank, World Health Organization (WHO)
Projected Job Growth	See the Future Growth section for trends in the industry

What is a Global Health Advisor?

A global health advisor is a public health subject-matter expert who offers advice to improve worldwide public health activities. They integrate research, regulations, policies, and actions in an organization's public health initiatives. They are employed in public, private, and non-profit international healthcare organizations and government agencies. They either work for one organization or work as a consultant for multiple healthcare agencies.[66]

Sample Case

Dr. Don Eliseo Lucero-Prisno III received his Doctor of Medicine degree from the University of the Philippines in 1997. He did not pursue a clinical specialization. Instead, he went into Global Health. He stated:

> I knew that I was going into medicine because I was very much interested in the field of health and development. I was exposed to many health issues when I was growing up – having a grandfather who died of lung cancer without access to medication and health services – and it opened my eyes to challenges in the healthcare field. Right after medical school, I joined a national program funded by the European Union. I was assisting in a national project because there was an increasing prevalence of HIV/AIDS cases at that time. When the project was finished, I worked for the Philippine government for five years. I was in health research management. I did not do any residency or clinical work or specialization.[67]

Dr. Don was recruited to work as Country Director for Access Health International in the Philippines. He shared:

> It is a senior-level management position that requires a vast knowledge of health systems. I have a postgraduate degree in health economics and research. It is easy for me to think of a scenario and provide advice. It is like working for a think tank. I provide the best strategies to reach a goal. Whether there are increasing HIV/AIDS or COVID-19 trends, by using different paradigms, I come up with programs.[67]

Roles and Responsibilities

Global health advisors are responsible for diagnosing, monitoring, and evaluating healthcare systems for problems and strategizing solutions to global health issues. They implement programs designed to improve general health. Dr. Don noted:

> As a more senior person within the organization, I advise the juniors on projects. I also advise the government. Currently, we are strengthening the health system of the Philippines. Daily, we look at programs following a program calendar. We are looking at achieving different timetables for the activities. We have goals and, eventually, we implement different aspects. For example, how can we improve the service delivery network to implement the Philippines' Universal Health Coverage? We also produce research. For example, how should a network deliver non-communicable disease services within Metro Manila? How is the current network being delivered?[67]

Global health advisors oversee and connect government and non-government health communities to public health programs. They coordinate programs with all constituents and partners to link and match public health resources with the local community's needs.[66] Some programs are geared for preventing and controlling communicable and vector-borne diseases such as health hazards management, sexually transmitted disease control, and immunization. Other programs decelerate drug and alcohol abuse and improve mental health treatment. There are programs that facilitate public health concerns through education, research, policymaking, and services. This includes community health, family planning, migrant health, and workforce management to underserved and at-risk communities, to name a few.[68] Dr. Don explained some of the projects he is currently overseeing in the Philippines:

> We have a tuberculosis project. We also have a World Health Organization and World Bank project, where we strengthen the health system by setting up strategies to assist in the Universal Health Coverage. We also develop proposals. We must craft proposals because there will be international donors who will request them. We have partner organizations like the World Surgical Foundation and the Philippine College of Surgeons. They are interested in strengthening the surgery aspect of the health system.[67]

Skills, Education, Certification, and Training

Most healthcare organizations prefer global health advisors have a Master of Public Health degree or a global health educational background. Additionally, candidates with experience or special knowledge in healthcare policy and law, healthcare systems, and healthcare economics receive more offers than their counterparts. For example, Dr. Don furthered his education to improve his expertise and prepare for a global health career. He said:

> I decided that I would need extra academic degrees, and the best way to hone my skills was to go abroad. I was interested in health policy, so I earned my Master of Public Health degree at the Royal Tropical Institute in Amsterdam. I got a scholarship and earned my Master of Science in Health Economics, Policy and Law in Global Health degree at Erasmus University in Rotterdam. Then, I earned my PhD in Global Health at Cardiff University in the UK. All the while, I was always focusing on health and development. [67]

To become a successful global health advisor, you need to sharpen your program management, verbal and written communication, problem-solving, and critical thinking skills. It is also vital to synthesize non-healthcare concepts such as urban development, poverty, and sanitation with healthcare concepts. Dr. Don explained:

> You accumulate skills, you accumulate knowledge. You innovate and, eventually, you also accumulate responsibility. You keep on moving forward. You keep on accepting more challenges. [67]

Pros and Cons

Some advantages to becoming a global health advisor are:

1. Global health is a gratifying career. As a global health advisor coordinating health program management, you can successfully implement programs that impact millions of people.

2. Your clinical experience boosts your resume. A survey completed by USAID found that 66% of project directors believed that a Master of Public Health degree and global health educational programs do not adequately prepare the students who possess no clinical skills.[69] Hence, clinical experience will boost your candidacy for a job compared to those without it.

3. Travel for conferences and meetings. This career involves plenty of traveling. Traveling may be domestic (in your own country visiting the field to check on the feasibility or coordination of a local program) or it could be international (attending international conferences, events, and sometimes international programs).

4. Work with industry leaders. You will get the chance to work with thought leaders and key stakeholders in your prospective locality or country. You will work with changemakers to provide support, guidance, and even financial backing to your programs.

5. Work with a diverse community. Most of your programs will touch thousands, if not millions, of lives. To make this a reality, you will work closely with local members of the community. These coordinators know the community by heart, and it is essential to have their support and participation. Some programs will allow you to work with multiple organizations.

Some challenges to becoming a global health advisor are:

1. Mandated tenure decreases job security. Most international healthcare organizations have tenure mandates that allow global health advisors to work for only a year or two. On a brighter note, you can jump from one healthcare organization to another. This varies your experience.

2. Competitive. Most graduates of the Master of Public Health with a Global Health Concentration will search for the same job. It is vital to find your niche. Dr. Don advised:

> Find an area where you are the only specialist. For me, it is maritime health. The Philippines has the greatest number of seafarers. I got interested in it because no one was interested. I did my master's and PhD theses on maritime health. You keep on doing a lot of work in that field and, eventually, you get recognized. You can do many things but have a special area and a special focus that will make you stand out from the rest. Because I am the only specialist in this field, I sit in on shipping company meetings to provide advice on repatriation of seafarers. I get interviewed by the media. I am the only specialist they will call on. So, you keep on receiving emails. That is one technique. [67]

3. Few entry-level jobs. New graduates are seldom considered for entry-level or mid-level positions due to competition with experienced global health workers vying for those positions. A study by Keralis et al. analyzed 1,007 global health job vacancies from 127

international healthcare organizations from November 2015 to March 2016. Their results showed that 40% were for subject-matter experts, 20% for program directors, 16% for managers, 13.6% for mid-levels, and only 9.8% for entry-level positions.[70]

Future Growth

There are mixed feelings on future growth of the global health advisory role. There are a few entry-level and mid-level positions for recent graduates of international public health programs. While the supply of the positions is limited, global training programs continue to produce graduates every semester. The supply is outpacing the demand.[70]

On the other hand, an article from Johns Hopkins Bloomberg School of Public Health stated that the long-term outlook is bright for new graduates seeking public health jobs. They discussed that COVID-19 has placed global public health safety in the minds of international and domestic governments. Even with the economic downturn for most countries, federal funding delays, and maxed out emergency budgets, the author of the article is hopeful for the global health sector's future growth.[71]

Now What?

1. If this career has piqued your interest, the first consideration is how much education you will need to move forward. It is highly recommended you complete a Master of Public Health degree. Completing a Master of Science in Health Economics, Policy and Law degree will be a bonus. You can widen your search to include international schools. Some programs may have scholarships that would cover your tuition.

2. Find a niche. It is essential to realize that finding an untapped sector will do wonders for your career in global health. After finding your area of interest, you need to learn as much as you can about this specialty. Consume as much information as possible about your niche. Read books and articles. Listen to webinars and go to conferences. After you consume, it is time to create. Write an article for an industry journal, start a webinar, be a speaker at a conference to educate colleagues about your specialty. Get your name recognized in that niche.

3. Network with someone from your prospective organization. The best resource is LinkedIn. Search for the company name in the search bar, and filter by the "People" icon. This will

give you a comprehensive list of possible connections. Send a "Connect" invite and always "Add a Note." The "Add a Note" section is a free tool on LinkedIn. Write a short paragraph on why you are reaching out. Here is an example:

> Hello Sir/Madam,
>
> I am looking to expand my connection in the field of global health. I saw that you work for XYZ organization. I would love to connect, hear about your experiences, and gain advice on how to leverage my medical degree for this career. Can we do a virtual coffee?
>
> Sincerely,
> Your name

Your goal is to give your time to get their time. Set up a Zoom virtual coffee. Hear their story. Then, share your story and what you are looking for. Genuinely get to know the person. Keep in touch with them every month. You will create a lasting impression and be first on their call list when there are future openings within their organization.

About Dr. Don

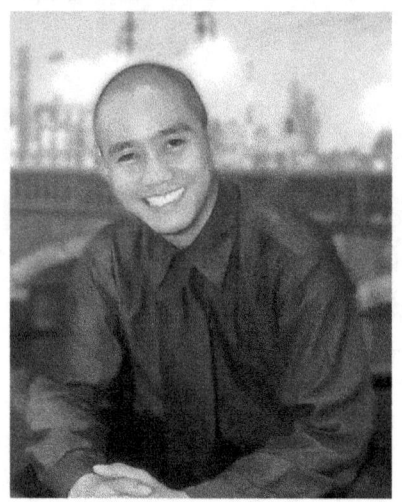

Don Eliseo Lucero-Prisno III, MD, PhD, MPH, MSc earned his Doctor of Medicine degree from the University of the Philippines, Manila, the Philippines in 1997, a Master of Public Health degree from Royal Tropical Institute in Amsterdam, Netherlands in 2004, and a Diploma in Social Science Research Methods from Cardiff University, UK in 2005. He also received a PhD degree from Cardiff University, UK in 2014, a Master of Science in Health Economics, Policy and Law degree from Erasmus University, Rotterdam, Netherlands in 2015, and a Certificate in Professional Studies in Learning and Teaching in Higher Education from the University of Liverpool, UK in 2018.

Professionally, he was a University Instructor in Psychology and Behavioral Sciences in De La Salle University, Manila, the Philippines from 1990-1992, National STD/HIV/AIDS Coordinator for the European Union STD/HIV/AIDS Capability Building Program of the Philippines with the Department of Health, Manila, the Philippines from 1997-1998, and Senior Science Research Specialist for the Philippine Council for Health Research and Development from 1999-2003. He became Health and HIV/AIDS Advisor for the Philippine Seafarers Assistance Program with the International Committee on Seafarers Welfare of Rotterdam, Netherlands from 2003-2005. He also completed his Nippon Foundation Research Fellowship at Cardiff University, UK in 2009. He then became Lecturer for Public Health for the University of Liverpool from 2010-2019 and Associate Professor of Global Health for the Xi'an Jiaotong-Liverpool University, Suzhou, Jiangsu Province, China from 2014-2019.

Currently, he works as Country Director for ACCESS Health International in Manila, Philippines, Research Associate in Global Health for the Global Health Institute (Wuhan University, China), Tutor of Economics of Global Health Policy (London School of Hygiene and Tropical Medicine, UK), Professorial Lecturer in International Health (University of the Philippines), Honorary Consultant for the College of Health Systems Management (Naresuan University, Thailand), Adjunct Professor (La Sapientia Catholic University, Congo), Visiting Professor in Global Health College of Public Health (Taipei Medical University, Taiwan) and Associate Research Fellow for the School of Social Sciences (Cardiff University, UK). Non-academically, he is Founder and Managing Director of Global Health Focus and Managing Editor for the BMC Global Health Research and Policy Journal.

In his spare time Dr. Don loves to play sports, travel, and engage in civic work and outreach programs.

Chapter 9

Health Informatics Specialist

Overview

Job Title	Health Informatics Specialist / Health Informatician / Health Information Systems Specialist / Medical Informatics Specialist / Clinical Informatics Specialist / Biomedical Informatics Specialist / Health Informatics Consultant / Health Informatics Analyst
Salary Range	Average annual income in the US: $74,177. Ranges from $61,000 (10th percentile) to $89,000 (90th percentile)[72]
Education	Minimum of bachelor's or master's degree in health informatics. Recommended certifications in the US: • CPHIMS (from HIMSS) • RHIA (from AHIMA) Recommended certifications (from FEDIP) in the UK: • Practitioner • Senior Practitioner • Advanced Practitioner • Leading Practitioner
Training	On-the-job training available
Skills/Talents	Patient care, medical records, project management, strategy and planning skills, data management skills, proficiency in IT[1]
Sample Companies	Ascension Health, Baptist Health, Booz Allen Hamilton, Boston Group, Cigna, Community Healthcare Network, Deaconess Health System, Dignity Health, Foundation Medicine, Health Services Advisory Group, Mayo Clinic, Tri-County Health Department, Winchester Hospital
Projected Job Growth	Approximately 9% increase in the US from 2018-2028[72]

What is a Health Informatics Specialist?

Health informatics is the storage, interpretation, and management of health information technology. It primarily uses electronic health records to design, develop, implement, and adopt IT-based solutions for health care service delivery improvement.[73,74] A health informatics specialist applies and manages health information technology to improve health outcomes. They work for the government, hospitals, long-term care facilities, mental health facilities, rehab facilities, outpatient clinics, insurance companies, medical device companies, private software companies, and other healthcare delivery service companies.

There are several sub-specialties in the health informatics field, namely bioinformatics, public health informatics, and clinical and nursing informatics. Translational bioinformatics creates bridges between fundamental biological concepts and clinical informational systems. These subspecialists develop processes and approaches for biomedical sciences. Public health informatics, on the other hand, tackles characterization, evaluation, and refinement of healthcare services, products, and techniques to improve quality, safety, and patient outcomes. Clinical and nursing informatics delves into acquisition, storage, retrieval, and use of health information technology to improve clinical decision support systems and refine clinical processes in the context of improving patient care. Public health informatics deals with large scale population health outcomes, while clinical informatics deals with individualized patient outcomes.[75,76]

Sample Case

Dr. Ismat Mohd Sulaiman earned her Doctor of Medicine degree from Universiti Kebangsaan in Malaysia in 2006. She also completed a Master of Science in Health Informatics degree from Karolinska Institutet, Stockholm University, Sweden in 2016. She explored alternatives to working as a clinician and found the health informatics field. She stated:

> My friends were going for master's programs to become specialists. I thought about what was out there on the other side of the clinical field. I wanted to explore how to support patient care and clinical conditions. So, I applied to work at the Health Informatics Centre in the Ministry of Health. I asked my boss to give me a six-month trial period. I told her that if I felt this was a place where I could contribute, I would stay. Otherwise, I would go back to clinical work because I loved my clinical job. After three months in the Health Informatics Centre, I knew it was where my heart belonged.[77]

Roles and Responsibilities

A health informatics specialist is primarily an administrative support professional. Some of the roles and responsibilities of a health informatics specialist include implementing and maintaining electronic health records, developing and implementing new methods of cataloging and managing patient information, managing databases, building new systems, testing established systems, analyzing and leveraging data sets, and planning for organizational integration.[76,78,79]

Dr. Ismat shared one of her national projects on establishing a digital health data warehouse. Her national project was instrumental in disease surveillance of COVID-19. She stated:

> Data warehouses are usually localized. Some are at universities and some are located at a municipal or state level. We needed to establish a data warehouse at a national level to examine the population of the public and private healthcare sector. Other than the basic reporting, we included other components, like a geographic information system to manage health systems for surveillance of disease. We also extended our data warehouse to include artificial intelligence techniques. This is completed through text processing to generate and pull-out information from clinical notes.
>
> I also train other health informatics specialists on how to use the system, generate reports, and create visualization. For example, when the director of the hospital asks for information, can you produce it? A health informatics specialist reduces workload because with the information they produce, administrators no longer key into MS Excel, calculate, and create a chart. We have a system database so that the data collection process is automated.[77]

Skills, Education, Certification, and Training

Dr. Ismat explored her passion for data and informatics. She joined the Health Informatics Center before receiving her master's degree in health informatics. She stated:

> I learned how to manage healthcare data and how to create reports and visualize those reports so stakeholders could act upon them. I learned how systems were developed and about standards in health informatics to make sure systems were integrated.[77]

Generally, the key to becoming a health informatics specialist is building a strong foundation of informatics education and clinical experience. Health informatics specialists take courses for a certification or degree to advance in their field. There are several options for education in this career field: Bachelor of Science in Health Informatics, Bachelor of Science in Business – Information Technology Management, Bachelor of Information Technology or Master of Science in Health Informatics, Master of Informational Systems, Master of Health Informatics, or Master of Nursing Informatics.[75] To find a reputable program in the US, check for Commission on Accreditation for Health Informatics and Health Information Management Education (CAHIIM) accredited schools from their website. Like Dr. Ismat, it is possible to get sponsorship for your advanced degree from your healthcare sector. She stated that when she went to study, she was sponsored by the government and Karolinska Institut in return for an agreed upon contract of employment service.

After receiving a minimum of two years of education, health informatics specialists can be credentialed in their field to boost their credibility. This is not mandatory, but highly advised. In the US, the American Health Information Management Association (AHIMA) offers credentials as a Registered Health Information Administrator (RHIA). The Healthcare Information and Management Society, Inc (HIMSS) provides certification as a Certified Professional in Health Information and Management Systems (CPHIMS). In the UK, the Federation for Informatics Professionals in Health and Social Care (FEDIP) offers professional registrations as Practitioner, Senior Practitioner, Advanced Practitioner, and Leading Practitioner based on FEDIP Standards of Professional Competence.[73] Dr. Ismat explained:

> The hard skills, those are all in textbooks. The soft skills, like how to negotiate, listen, and talk need to be developed to understand the clinicians and stakeholders' requirements and relay that information correctly to IT engineers. Be willing to learn from your mistakes. It is okay to make a mistake. Admit it, and then improve.[77]

Pros and Cons

Some advantages to becoming a health informatics specialist are:

1. Health informatics is a new industry. In the US, the Health Information Technology for Economic and Clinical Health (HITECH) Act was signed into law as part of the American Recovery and Reinvestment Act of 2009. This law's primary aim was to encourage the adoption and meaningful use of electronic health records and health information technology.[78] Additionally, the European Union enacted the Directive 2011/24/EU that

boosted access to electronic health records anywhere in Europe.[79] The need for health information management professionals is vital to this process.

2. Diversification in the healthcare technology industry. Your progress with health information management can be coupled with other emerging industries such as data analytics, machine learning, and artificial intelligence. Combing these concepts in practice is in its infancy. There is substantial room for growth and development.

Some challenges to becoming a health informatics specialist are:

1. Finding an entry-level job is tough. Even though it is an entry-level position, most entry-level jobs in this field require experience. It is a two-edged sword when you are new and do not have experience. One way to circumnavigate this is to get group or supervised experience. Dr. Ismat advised:

> Try to get involved in small projects. Find a problem that you experienced in your clinic or hospital and offer yourself to the hospital director to solve this problem. It builds your CV and it gives you some experience. Later, if you do decide that this is your thing, then plan for advanced education.[77]

2. This career requires an investment. You will need to enroll in an advanced degree and complete a certification to begin in this field. Expect to invest $30,000-$40,000 for two years in an accredited program before landing your first job.

3. Practice makes perfect. You will be learning numerous technical skills in your courses. This can be overwhelming for a newcomer, but be vigilant about your passion. Practice, practice, practice.

Future Growth

Health informatics is a new and groundbreaking healthcare profession. Health information technology such as electronic health record systems, online patient portals, and health applications is a popular field. CNBC reported that healthcare providers, globally, are spending over $100 billion each year on health information technology.[80] Investments in health information technology will propel this industry into creating more data and information. This will increase the demand for professionals in this field to manage and leverage this information technology transformation. There is a projected job growth of approximately 9% in the US from 2018 to 2028.[72]

Now What?

1. Try your hand at an internal project. As mentioned earlier, find a problem in your current healthcare organization and volunteer to solve the problem. Here are some examples: Create an Excel spreadsheet of patients undergoing cardiac catherization in Quarter 4 (September to December) and analyze their risk factors. Create an Excel spreadsheet of patients who have completed their colonoscopy in the year 2020 and examine their demographics.

2. Try your hand with external databases. If internal projects are unavailable, try external datasets. Kaggle.com provides datasets across different industries. Find a problem in the healthcare field and search for relevant dataset within your chosen topic. Work on the problem to determine an optimal solution. This exercise will provide you with real world experience.

3. More exploration. If you are unable to find projects, try exploring through course offerings. Take a health informatics or health analytics course through Udemy.com or Coursera.com. Udemy courses cost an average of $12.99 on their sale dates, while Coursera ranges from free to $300, depending on whether or not you want a signed certificate of completion.

4. Network with health informatics professionals. Search for "Health Informatics" in the LinkedIn search bar. Filter your search by the "People" icon. Send a "Connect" invite and always "Add a Note." The "Add a Note" section is a free tool on LinkedIn. Write a short paragraph on why you are reaching out. Here is an example:

> Hello Sir/Madam,
>
> I am looking to pivot to the healthcare technology field. I saw that you work for XYZ organization. I would love to connect and hear about your experiences. Can we do a virtual coffee?
>
> Sincerely,
> Your name

Set up a Zoom virtual coffee. Hear their story. Then, share your story and what you are looking for. Keep in touch with them every month. You will create a lasting impression and be first on their call list when there are future openings within their organization.

5. Get proper education and training. When you are steadfast about your decision to proceed to health informatics, find an accredited program. Accreditation reviews are spearheaded by the Commission on Accreditation for Health Informatics and Information Management Educations (CAHIIM) in the US and the Canadian Health Information Management Association (CHIMA) in Canada. To search, go to the organization's website.

6. Take the certification exams. In the US, keep in mind that you cannot sit for these certification exams if you have not completed the educational component of health information management from an accredited program. There are two certifying organizations in the US: AHIMA offers an RHIA certification and HIMSS offers CPHIMS certification. FEDIP offers professional registrations as Practitioner, Senior Practitioner, Advanced Practitioner, and Leading Practitioner in the UK.

About Dr. Ismat

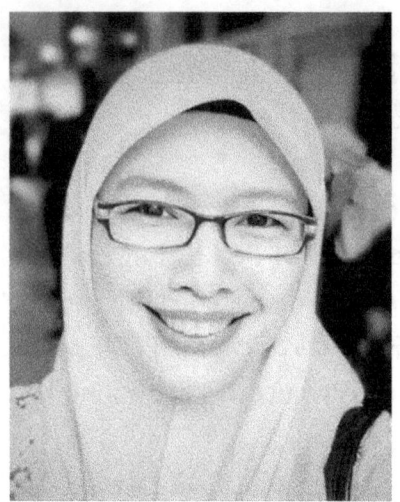

Ismat Mohd Sulaiman, MD, MSc is a clinician and health informatician. She earned her Doctor of Medicine degree from Universiti Kebangsaan in Malaysia in 2006. She also completed a Master of Science in Health Informatics from Karolinska Institutet, Stockholm University, Sweden in 2016. Dr. Ismat wrote and published her thesis, *Mapping Cardiology Registry to SNOWMED CT: A comparative study between Malaysia and Sweden*. She is currently a doctoral student for the Social and Preventive Medicine Department, Faculty of Medicine at the University of Malaya in Malaysia.

Currently, she is Senior Principal Assistant Director UD54 for the Health Informatics Centre, Ministry of Health in Putrajaya, Malaysia. She is Malaysia's nominated representative in the International Health Terminology Standards Development Organization (IHTSDO) / SNOMED International. Two of her most significant projects include being Project Lead for MyHarmony and implementing an Executive Information System within the Hospital Information System throughout Malaysia. Dr. Ismat has received several awards including the Excellent Service Awards (twice) from the Ministry of Health Malaysia (Anugerah Perkhidmatan Cemerland) in 2012 and 2017.

In her spare time she works on edible gardening while thinking about improving health care — one piece of information at a time.

Chapter 10

Health Insurance Advisor

Overview

Job Title	Health Insurance Advisor / Health Insurance Broker
Salary Range	Average annual income in the US: $50,940. Ranges from $28,000 (10th percentile) to $125,000 (90th percentile)[81]
Education	Pass the State Licensing Examination
Training	On-the-job training available in some companies
Skills/Talents	Analytical skills, initiative, self-confidence, communication skills
Sample Companies	Independent brokerage firms: Hub International, Marsh and McLennan Cos Inc, USHealth Advisors Captive health insurance firms: Aetna, Blue Cross Blue Shield, Cigna, Humana, UnitedHealthcare
Projected Job Growth	Approximately 5% increase in the US from 2019-2029[81]

What is a Health Insurance Advisor?

A health insurance advisor is a licensed health benefits professional who helps individuals research, set up, buy, and manage health insurance plans from the beginning to the end of the process. Their main objective is to educate and advise individuals on health insurance plan selection so they can make an educated decision.[82]

The target populations for health insurance advisors vary, but mainly they are small business owners and self-employed professionals. They may be new small business owners figuring out health benefits on their own after being dropped by their employer's insurance, or they may be established, self-employed professionals who are looking to change health insurance. The health insurance advisor provides insight into different options to find an insurance plan that best suits each situation.

Sample Case

Noor Afsa Ali, MBBS, MPH, CPH, GCIP earned her Bachelor of Medicine and Bachelor of Surgery degree from Kumudini Women's Medical College in Bangladesh in 2013. She pivoted from medicine and became a health insurance advisor. She explained:

> After medical school I moved back to the States, got married, and started a family. The next step entailed passing the United States Medical Licensing Exams (USMLE), getting into a good residency program, and completing residency. I dedicated two years of my life to studying exclusively for the Step Exams. I did not do anything else. Unfortunately, I did not pass. I failed by three points. After dedicating two years of my life and not getting any traction, I was spiraling into a mental state of depression, loss of self-esteem, and a lack of self-worth. In Bangladesh, I was a superstar. I was completing surgeries. The stark difference in performance took a mental toll on me. So, I decided it was time to capitalize on my other skills and asked myself how could I utilize these other skills to pivot into an alternative career. I did not want to waste more years of my life just chasing ghosts.
>
> When you go to medical school, everyone has this expectation. It is important to keep in mind that life never goes as planned, and that's okay. You reach a point where you cannot care so much about what everybody else says, and you must figure out your own best solution. What is good for you? This

might not work for your family, or your next-door neighbor, and that is okay. It is okay to fail as long as you get back up and find something that works. It is okay to not go the traditional route of medicine and find your way in this world. Just do you.[83]

Roles and Responsibilities

In the US, before the Affordable Care Act was passed in 2008, individuals qualified for health insurance according to their health status. To capitalize on clinical knowledge, it was easier to evaluate someone according to their health and offer different health insurance plans.[83] Dr. Noor stated:

> I ask my clients questions regarding their health evaluation for medical underwriting purposes. Daily, people come to me looking for health insurance. They are young, healthy, and barely go to the doctor. They have no chronic illnesses and take no regular prescription medications. They need a plan to cover them, specifically. Most health insurance plans in the market are costly, with high premiums and high deductibles. However, a health insurance advisor can qualify this type of client for health-based programs. Self-employed professionals and small businesses also qualify for these plans. Once qualified, a health insurance advisor can walk through the enrollment process via screen share to get the client the best insurance reflective of their health.[83]

Skills, Education, Certification, and Training

Health insurance advisors are licensed and regulated by state insurance departments. The Florida exam is called 2-15 Life, Health, and Annuities and administered by the Florida Department of Financial Services. There are courses (60-120 hours) specifically geared to help you pass this exam. Every state has its own set of laws, limitations, exclusions, and products offered. Health insurance advisors are required to complete continuing education to renew their licenses.

To become a successful health insurance advisor, it is crucial to have an entrepreneurial spirit. You should be self-driven and motivated with a growth mindset. Dr. Noor asserted:

> Physicians, even having attended medical school for one semester, are often oriented toward performance, achievement, competition, and wanting to be the best. Health insurance advisors share these traits but, like physicians,

they must also have an innate desire to help other people. Then, everything falls into place.[83]

Health insurance advising is a business venture. You are running your own business and your success is dependent on effort put forth. Most companies will give you the tools to start your own business, but growing your business depends on your hard work and creativity. You can market your business on different social media platforms. You can provide medical education to your prospective clients. You can give workshops to increase your credibility and establish rapport with possible clients. The sky is the limit with the variety of work that could come with this career.

Pros and Cons

Some advantages to becoming a health insurance advisor are:

1. There is unlimited earning potential. Health insurance advisors fall under two earning categories: captive and independent. Captive health insurance advisors receive a combination of salary and commission. This career professional often works with one specific health insurance carrier.[84] Independent health insurance advisors often work for an insurance brokerage firm that sells numerous health insurance plans. Dr. Noor elaborated:

   > As an independent health insurance advisor, my career is a commission-only job. There is no capitation on earnings on a commission-only job. You can make more money as a health insurance advisor than you could ever make being a salaried employee with a W-2 corporate job.[83]

2. You can have passive income. It took Dr. Noor two years (beyond taking a quarter off for pregnancy and delivery and another quarter off for research in Australia) to have a comfortable residual income. She considered her career trajectory slow compared to her peers. Dr. Noor explained:

   > I am at a stage in my career where I have a substantial monthly residual income coming in, which means whether I work or not, the commissions I get from my clients help me maintain my lifestyle. I can just take my hands off the wheel. My business is self-sustaining, it is thriving, and I do not have be so hands-on.[83]

3. There is a minimal barrier to entry. To become a Licensed Health Insurance Advisor, you must pass a state licensing exam. Often, this career has a fast-rising trajectory where you do not have to get another degree to make a lot of money. There is little to no overhead cost for starters.

4. There is excellent flexibility. Health insurance advisors can work from home and be their own boss. This is a family-friendly alternative. Dr. Noor reported that her work is entirely virtual. She can care for her baby and take client calls in the evening.

5. There is stability and security in this employment. Insurance is not going anywhere. It has been around for centuries. It will be essential for as long as the community needs education in understanding health benefits. During the recession, insurance is more stable than other fields because individuals will always need protection for their health risks.[84]

6. You are helping people. Dr. Noor stated:

    > It is very fulfilling because you are helping clients who have no idea how to navigate such a complicated industry. I get the same level of reward and gratitude as my clients. A health insurance plan can have zero deductibles and no co-pays. It's such a good feeling, especially when a customer refers me to someone else. I am in the stage of my career where I do not make outbound phone calls. I have referrals calling me for my services. It makes me feel so accomplished.[83]

7. You work for your client for free. The client does not directly pay your commission. Instead, the commission comes from the health insurance plan the client signs up with and you receive a portion of the client's monthly premium. Hence, your commission is not limited to the first year. You get paid as long as the insurance plan for that client is in effect.

Some challenges to becoming a health insurance advisor are:

1. Client acquisition can be challenging in the beginning. You will start your business by cold calling clients. It will take some time to build a clientele through cold calls and outbound calls. But, with vigilance and conviction, a health insurance advisor with little to no experience can achieve financial success relatively quickly. Once you have a good referral program in place, you can build your business through your previous clients' referrals.[84]

2. The sales process can be daunting. Yes, this career involves advising and selling individualized health insurance plans. Health insurance advisors are responsible for providing knowledge

and educating the client about the best individualized health insurance plan to suit their needs and budget. Also, to get paid, you must walk the client through the health insurance enrollment process. For a beginner with no sales background, this can be a challenge. However, most companies will provide you guidance and training through the sales process.

Future Growth

The future trend and growth in this market involves no ceilings and no capitations. According to the US Bureau of Labor Statistics, approximately 50% of the insurance workforce will retire in 2028.[85] There is an estimated 5% growth in the US from 2019 to 2029.[81] Employment growth is more robust for independent health insurance advisors than captive health insurance advisors. Most companies rely on insurance brokerage firms to help them control costs.

Now What?

1. Research the state licensing exam for your state. Once you have decided to pursue this career, the first step is to research and learn about the licensure exam. Keywords in Google.com include "Life, Health, and Annuities Examination." Familiarize yourself with the examination components.

2. Take a prep course before taking the exam. Again, search in Google.com for courses to prepare you for the licensure examination. Often, classes take 60-120 hours to complete.

3. Find an insurance brokerage partner. If you choose to be an independent health insurance advisor, then partner with insurance brokerage organizations. If you decide to be a captive health insurance advisor, find an insurance plan that suits your values. Some examples are Blue Cross Blue Shield, UnitedHealthcare, Aetna, Humana, and Cigna. These organizations walk you through the process. They provide tools and resources to land your first and future clients. They have access to contact lists for cold calling as you begin your business. They also train you on how to talk insurance.

4. Pass the state licensing exam and start with success in mind. In as little as 3-4 months, you can launch a new career and start making a good income. The first couple of phone calls can provoke anxiety, but you will do better with practice and repetition. Once you gain your bearings, subsequent phone calls will become easier. You will shine and you will succeed in this field.

About Dr. Noor

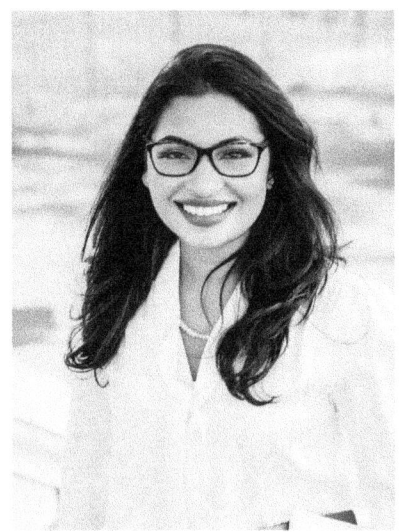

Noor Afsa Ali, MBBS, MPH, CPH, GCIP earned her Bachelor of Medicine and Bachelor of Surgery degree from Kumudini Women's Medical College, Bangladesh in 2013. She also completed her Master of Public Health degree with a concentration in Global Health Practice from the University of South Florida, USA in 2019. She earned a Graduate Certification in Public Health from the National Board of Public Health Examiners in 2019 and a Certification in Infection Control and Prevention from the University of South Florida in 2019. She received the Most Outstanding Member of the Junior Chamber International in Bangladesh in 2013 and the Most Outstanding Agent in Leadership from USHealth Advisor, US in 2018.

Currently, Dr. Noor is a Licensed Health Insurance Advisor for USHealth Advisors. She handles sales of health and life insurance and annuities in 30 states from the Florida Department of Financial Services.

Her other interests include research in women's reproductive health, maternal and child health, mom-preneurship, reading fantasy fiction, and traveling with her family experiencing food and culture around the world.

CHAPTER 11

Home Health Care Continuum

Overview

Job Title	Home Health Nurse / Home Health Clinical Manager / Home Health Supervisor / Director of Patient Care Services / Executive Director
Salary Range	Home Health Registered Nurse average annual salary in the US: $79,405. Ranges from $40,000 (10th percentile) to $122,500 (90th percentile)[86]
Education	Bachelor of Science in Nursing degree required, Registered Nurse licensure from your respective state
Training	On-the-job training for home health nurse is available in most companies
Skills/Talents	Clinical, nursing, organizational, and driving skills
Sample companies	Amedisys Home Health Care, Aveanna Healthcare, Bayada, Brookdale Senior Living Inc, Care UK Limited, Extendicare Inc, Genesis Healthcare Corp, Kindred Healthcare, Maxim Healthcare Services, Senior Care Centers of America, Sompo Holdings Inc
Projected Job Growth	Approximately 7.9% increase in the US from 2020-2027. The home health industry is forecasted to value $525.6 billion by 2027[87]

What is the Home Health Care Continuum?

Home health nursing is the delivery of medical care to patients in the patient's home. Home health nursing aims to foster patient safety at home, avoid hospitalization, and help patients return to their maximum functional level.[86] The home health nurse works directly in a home setting providing clinical patient care. Other positions in the home health care continuum are mainly non-clinical – administrative, supervisory, and executive in nature – and include home health clinical manager, home health supervisor, director of patient care services, and executive director. This later positions will be discussed in more detail later in the chapter.

Sample Case

Dr. Cezar Cunanan received his medical and nursing degrees from Our Lady of Fatima University, Philippines. He pivoted from practicing as a medical doctor and pursued a career in nursing in California, USA. Currently, Dr. Cezar is Executive Director of a home health agency.

Dr. Cezar explained that home health is an integrative, multidisciplinary approach needing a care team of licensed clinicians for nursing, physical therapy, occupational therapy, speech, social work, and home health assistance.[88]

Home health nurses work under home health agencies that provide rosters of patients to care for. Patients are discharged from hospitals, skilled nursing facilities, or long-term care facilities and cannot care for themselves. Patients vary to include the elderly with chronic conditions, those with mental illnesses, pediatric patients with debilitating diseases, and those who are recovering from surgery. Dr. Cezar's home health agency mainly works with elderly patients. He stated:

> The patients I care for average 65 to 70 years old. These patients either live by themselves, live with a family member, or have a hired caregiver. Some cannot live alone in their own home, so they stay in an assisted living facility or an adult living community.

> When I first applied for nursing jobs with an MD degree, I found that it can be a plus, but it can also work against you. Some employers think you are overqualified, and they are convinced you will eventually leave. But some employers also think that a medical background can help their organization. I was lucky because I was backed up by a friend who vouched for me.[88]

Dr. Cezar started his nursing career as a registered nurse (RN) field nurse for a California home health agency. He stated:

> RN field nurses are clinicians who visit patients in the home. I was also getting trained as a clinical manager in the office, which is a clinician who does the auditing for colleagues and their charts. I was lucky enough to train both in the field and in the office. I excelled in the office, working my way up from clinical manager to assistant director and then, finally, to a directorship role.[88]

Roles and Responsibilities

A home health nurse visits the patient's home to take vital signs, administer medication, draw blood, help with mobility, clean wounds, and educate patients about their conditions. The nurse visiting the patient in the home manages the patient's complete care. Nurses can work with one patient for several hours or work with multiple patients in one day.[87] Dr. Cezar explained that, generally, he had an average of 30 to 60 minutes to perform his visits and saw several patients in a day. New patients took more time than follow-up visits with established patients. Dr. Cezar explained:

> When I worked as a home health nurse, my day started with planning my route because I drove and had to anticipate what I was going to see in the home. Some patients had very nice homes. Some patients lived in dangerous neighborhoods. I needed to trust my instincts before entering a patient's home. When I entered a patient's home, I first had to identify the patient. I had to confirm that I was seeing the right patient and then introduced myself. Next, I found a place to safely put my bag. I had a home health bag containing restricted medications and supplies. I was responsible for having every needed basic supply I might require.
>
> When I started my visit, it was just like being in the clinic. I took vital signs and assessed the patient from head to toe. If I saw any deranged vitals, labs, equipment values, I had to know when to refer to the doctor and get new orders.[88]

Home health nurses also focus on new or established physician orders (assessments, blood, medications, or wound cleaning). Nurses report directly to clinical supervisors. Upon promotion, a home health nurse becomes a clinical supervisor/clinical manager.

Home health clinical supervisors are tasked with clinically assessing and supervising the delivery of home health nursing services. Although they are mainly administrative staff, they also perform home visits to evaluate and appraise whether nurses are practicing patient care consistent with agency policy and procedures. They oversee the nursing staff's work procedures and provide counseling, motivation, and mentorship when needed. Clinical supervisors also guide the nursing and support staff to ensure compliance and quality of clinical documentation. They conduct performance reviews. They also enhance operations through sufficient and efficient staffing.[89] Clinical supervisors report to clinical managers. Upon promotion, a clinical supervisor becomes a clinical manager.

Mainly administrative personnel, home health clinical managers are tasked with driving the home health agency forward. They are focused on day-to-day team management and effective patient care. They review, analyze, plan, coordinate, and manage the clinical team's activities to ensure quality home health care services to patients.[90] They also drive the productivity of required documentation and caseload. They select, train, and develop new clinical hires. They monitor, evaluate, and appraise established nurses and clinical supervisors. Clinical managers' report to the clinical director or executive director.[90,91] Upon promotion, a clinical manager becomes a director of patient care services/executive director.

The director of patient care services/executive director oversees the entire home health program. They are focused on overall agency performance. They work to plan, direct, and evaluate business operations and delivery of clinical services. They also provide leadership, guidance, and mentorship to clinical managers to meet the agency's goals and compliance requirements. As Executive Director, Dr. Cezar enumerated his responsibilities and what his day-to-day looks like:

> First, of course, I make sure we are abiding by state laws and regulations. I oversee the clinicians, making sure they know what is expected of them in the field and are executing their duties properly based on their licensure. When I arrive at the office, I have several items that I check in the first hour which will dictate my day. For example, I check how many admissions we have in a day. Then, who is to be discharged. Then, I must check my full-time employees. Are they carrying eight hours of work? Then, I assist the clinical supervisors and clinical managers with troubleshooting. Let us say you receive a call from a clinician that the patient is running a fever. Or another patient did not pick up the injection from the pharmacy. There is a lot of troubleshooting and delegation of work.[88]

Skills, Education, Certification, and Training

To begin as a home health nurse, you must complete a Bachelor of Nursing degree and pass the National Council Licensure Examination (NCLEX) to become licensed in your particular state. Experience is not necessary to start this career. Most home health agencies will train you to be a home health nurse. However, for the more senior positions, home health nursing experience is required.[88]

Some of the skills necessary to succeeding in this field are having good clinical and nursing skills. Dr. Cezar explained:

> As a home health nurse, you will apply your clinical skills. For example, you need to know the meaning of a BP of 100/90 – a narrow pulse pressure. What does this derangement of a vital sign mean? You must learn the value of reading and consistently learning to enhance your clinical and nursing skills. If you are not familiar with a certain medication, there are many apps out there to educate you. Look at the most common side effects, so if that medication appears again, next time you will know. You can put a face on that drug, and you will never forget it.[88]

Your nursing skills will be tested constantly during troubleshooting. Dr. Cezar relayed that it is essential to understand the limits of your license as a nurse. He stated:

> You need not panic when you encounter a problem. You deal with the problem and know when to ask for help. I think a good RN knows when to refer to the physician. And because doctors are so busy, and you do not often talk to the doctor – just the medical assistants or nurse practitioners – your report should be complete, concise, and brief.[88]

Pros and Cons

Some advantages of a career in home health care nursing are:

1. There are excellent career growth opportunities in a home health agency. With every year you work as a home health nurse, you get closer to promotion and growth. An average of 2.5 years of experience as a nurse can lend credibility and expertise for promotion – from home health nurse to clinical supervisor to clinical manager to clinical director to executive director.

2. Home health nursing is a fast-growing industry. As the population ages, the demand for home health nursing increases. See the future growth section for more details.

3. Flexibility. Your hours are not set from 9 a.m. to 5 p.m. You can schedule personal appointments as long as you complete eight hours a day. Also, there will be times when you are on call. For example, you are already home from visiting your last patient when one of your patients has an emergency. So, you must grab your medical bag, get back in your car, and visit the patient.

4. On-the-job training is available. Dr. Cezar stated:

> I do the hiring. I like hiring staff with no experience. I had no experience entering this field and somebody believed in me. So, I like molding people. New hires with no experience are like sponges. You tell them what you want to see in the field, and they follow your instruction. On the contrary, when clinicians have worked with several companies, there are good and bad aspects to that situation. They are experienced. They already know what to expect. They know how to troubleshoot. But, at the same time, there may be some bad habits to correct. They will always compare you with their previous companies. Each company is different. So, if you are working for an agency, make sure you abide by their policies.[88]

5. Independence. Depending on your perspective and character, this can be a positive or a negative. Though you have a team for support and guidance 24/7, you are the sole nurse during patient visits. You must be confident in your nursing skills, including phlebotomy.

6. You will work with different personalities among both patients and staff. Your patients will vary from those who do not want you to visit to those who will love your visits. Some will challenge your patience and composure, while there will be those who will make your day.

Some challenges of a career in home health care nursing are:

1. You will be driving a lot. A home health nurse is assigned patients by region. Your commute to a patient's home can take five minutes, 30 minutes, or one hour one way. Be prepared to drive through traffic and rush hour periods.

2. You spend a lot of time on documentation. There will be times where you work days and also nights to complete your documentation. There are documentation requirements you must meet to comply with state regulations and policies.

Future Growth

The majority of home health patients are elderly. According to the World Health Organization in 2019, the elderly population (aged 65 and above) was composed of 703 million persons worldwide. However, by 2050, the elderly population is projected to double to 1.5 billion persons. This expansive increase in the aging population will demand patient-centric home health services, which will drive the demand for home health nursing professionals. In the US, Medicare (the federal health program for patients 65 years old and over) is the largest payer of home health services.[87]

The global home health industry was valued at $281.8 billion dollars in 2019 and $303.6 billion dollars in 2020. It is expected to grow by 7.9% in the United States from 2020 to 2027. It is forecasted to value $525.6 billion by 2027.[87]

Now What?

1. Get your transcript evaluated. If this is the path you want to take, the first step is to complete a Bachelor of Nursing degree. As an International Medical Graduate, some of your courses will accelerate your process, so it is vital to have your credentials evaluated by a foreign education transcript evaluation organization. Examples of these organizations include American Association of Collegiate Registrars and Admissions Officers (AACRAO), Educational Credential Evaluators Inc, Educational Perspectives, Foundation of International Services Inc, International Credential Assessment Services of Canada, International Educational Research Foundation, and World Education Services Inc. Dr. Cezar used World Education Services Inc for his transcript evaluation.[88] After receiving an evaluation, your Bachelor of Science in Nursing four-year degree will often be decreased by approximately two years. There are even some accelerated programs that allow completion in a little over a year.

2. Research schools and apply. Now you are ready to Google schools and check their admission requirements. This is a meticulous process, but necessary to selecting a program that suits your journey. Be mindful of in-state versus out-of-state tuition differences. You may need to apply for government tuition assistance.

3. Take the state licensure examination. Unique sets of policies and regulations govern each state.

4. Find a home health agency in your area and apply.

About Dr. Cezar:

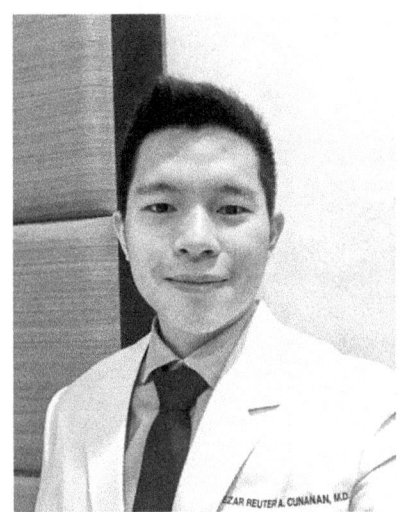

Cezar Reuter Cunanan, MD, RN received his Doctor of Medicine degree (2009-2013) and Bachelor of Science in Nursing degree (2003-2007) from Our Lady of Fatima University, Philippines. He is a Licensed Registered Nurse (RN) in California. He started as an RN Clinical Supervisor for Amity Home Health Care in Hayward, California (2013-2014). He, then, pivoted to become Clinical Supervisor for Golden Pacific Home Health in Alameda, California (2014). He became Assistant Director of Patient Care Services for the same organization (2014-2015). He then moved to Amedisys Home Health in Hayward, California as Clinical Manager (2017-2020) and Director of Operations/Administrator (2015-2017). He pivoted again to Executive Director/Administrator for Healthy Living at Home in San Jose, California (2020 to present).

Chapter 12

Medical Educator

Overview

Job Title	Medical Educator / Medical Education Consultant / Medical Education Advisor / Medical Education Specialist / Clinician Educator
Salary Range	Average annual income in the US: $75,530. Ranges from $51,000 (10th percentile) to $103,000 (90th percentile).[92] Average annual income in Australia: $240,000 AUD[93]
Education	There are no qualifications required for entry-level. Graduate Certificate and Master of Clinical Education degree are expected for senior levels
Training	On-the-job training available in some companies
Skills/Talents	Verbal and written communication skills, teaching skills, problem-solving and mentoring skills, teamwork, management skills at senior levels
Sample companies	Ann & Robert H. Lurie Children's Hospital of Chicago, AstraZeneca, Christus Health, Emerson Ecologics, Novasyte, Pfizer, Philips, Stanford University School of Medicine, The University of Texas Medical Branch, UCLA Health, University of California, Irvine School of Medicine, University of Pittsburgh School of Medicine, University of Southern California (USC) Keck School of Medicine, Virginia Commonwealth University (VCU) School of Medicine
Projected Job Growth	Approximately 13% increase in the US from 2019-2029[94]

What is a Medical Educator?

Medical educators are crucial in teaching and training medical students and junior doctors in hospitals, and medical and vocational institutions. They provide direction and expertise for planning, implementing, and evaluating medical education programs and curriculum. They aim to enhance the teaching, training, and learning culture within clinical fields.[95,96]

Sample Case

Rebecca Stewart, MBBS earned her Bachelor of Medicine and Bachelor of Surgery degree from the University of Queensland, Australia in 1996 and a Fellowship of the Royal Australian College of General Practitioners in 2001. She continues her medical practice as a General Practitioner (GP), yet the majority of her career is spent as Medical Education Consultant and National Clinical Lead for the Royal Australian College of General Practitioners. Dr. Bec stated:

> Until five years ago, I have worked in mainstream general practice. But as I forayed into my medical education career, I found it a bit tricky to juggle a comprehensive clinical practice and the associated paperwork, skills, and knowledge required for medical education. So I started narrowing my scope of practice. I have worked as a GP in a voluntary psychiatric hospital, practiced skin cancer medicine, and practiced oncology. At the moment, I'm working as a GP with a special interest in cardiology at Townsville University Hospital in Queensland, Australia. I think it is important as an educator to still have your finger on the pulse of what's happening clinically. It also produces great learning material to share with my colleagues who are learning general practice.[93]

Dr. Bec elaborated on her launch into medical education:

> I suppose it was having a family that convinced me to make the change. When I had my first daughter, I was trying to juggle full-time practice, a new baby, and sleepless nights. It became very tricky. I was tapped on the shoulder by a fellow GP working at the university who asked me if I wanted to be a tutor in family studies. The job was teaching 4th year medical students about the skills needed to manage a new baby and a new family. I had personal experience to fall back on. I used to take my daughter along to tutorials, which was great. I soon realized that working in an academic environment was fulfilling and offered me a work/life balance. It provided me reasonable control over my

work schedule, which I found great. I took on a more senior teaching role and cut back my GP clinical work to two days a week. I guess it just started from there.[93]

She explained how she progressed through her career as a medical educator:

For the most part, clinicians become health educators because they are referred by professional peers. Interestingly, a lot of clinicians underestimate their ability to teach, so they wait to be invited. Again, I was tapped to be Director of Education for a GP training organization. Initially, I just trained GPs in my local region, but my position now is GP training Australia-wide. I want to serve a community by ensuring that the doctors are competent and safe in their practice.[93]

Roles and Responsibilities

Medical educators research, create, develop, implement, and deliver educational materials. They guide and facilitate learning with clinical integration. They review and update educational programs to align with emerging topics and technologies. They collaborate with other medical educators to promote scholarship and teaching excellence.

As National Clinical Lead for a large and established membership and training organization in Australia, Dr. Bec enumerated her roles and responsibilities as a medical educator:

My day consists of lots of Zoom meetings, since staff members are distributed throughout Australia. There are rules and regulations for working and training in general practice mandated by the government which need to be followed. I spend quite a lot of time reviewing policy and legislation, making sure it is implemented appropriately. Generally, I plan and conduct research and evaluation, provide mentorship and professional development for my team members, and develop educational programs and match them to national and international curricula. I fill multiple representative roles on different committees and councils and I provide individualized advice for learners. My role involves significant problem-solving and risk mitigation.[93]

When asked about her current projects, Dr. Bec stated:

> I am very passionate about ensuring that education is high quality, yet affordable and have developed online courses. For example, I developed a curriculum-mapped study planning app to help doctors as they are studying, making sure they understand the breadth of general practice. I have developed a clinical reasoning module, using case studies, to explore methods of diagnostic and therapeutic reasoning. Lack of clinical reasoning skills is the most common reason doctors have difficulty passing their final exams. I am thinking about going back and doing a course in instructional design. I actively look for opportunities where I can support doctors. I want to bottle the key concepts in order to impact a greater number of people. I want to potentiate the effectiveness and dissemination of information and broaden the skills I can offer.[93]

Skills, Education, Certification, and Training

Medical doctors are committed to teaching and learning. Dr. Bec explained:

> There is an assumption in medicine that doctors teach. It is part of the Hippocratic Oath. But that does not mean doctors are good teachers. The first challenge is having the confidence in yourself to go down that path. It is also important to recognize the skill sets you need and actively seek opportunities to develop them.[93]

There is no mandatory education, certification, or training. The UK and Australia have created curriculum frameworks to professionalize the responsibility of medical educators. In the UK, they aim to demonstrate knowledge, skills, attitudes, and behaviors of those involved in a teaching role.[95] The International Association for Medical Education (AMEE) is the main body for medical education.[96] The Academy of Medical Educators (AoME) developed the Academy Professional Standards Framework in the UK. The aim of these standards is to advocate for professional development and demonstrate commitment among medical educators.[97]

In Australia, the Australian Curriculum Framework for Junior Doctors (ACF) teaches medical educators to plan, develop, and conduct teaching sessions for peers and juniors. They use varied approaches to group teaching, incorporate teaching into clinical work, and evaluate feedback on teaching skills.[95,98] In 2008, Queensland Health developed the Medical Education Registrar (MER) program to provide clinical education and training in Australia. This framework integrated critically-needed future teaching skills into specialty programs for junior doctors.[97]

Clinicians must possess good verbal and written communication skills. It is even more important as a medical educator. Good communication skills are crucial to working effectively as a team. Dr. Bec added that being a team player was vital to making sure you can perform in any role within the team.[93]

Pros and Cons

Some advantages to becoming a medical educator are:

1. Work/life balance. Most medical educators complete their responsibilities from 9 a.m. to 5 p.m., five days a week. Some roles need an additional one to three hours, especially when grading exams, papers, and projects. Often, this is a family-friendly career.

2. Some classes are online. With widespread online learning platforms accelerated by COVID-19, many courses are delivered online. This offers further flexibility to a medical educator's time and workload management.

3. Job security and stability. There is an increasing demand for medical educators, as most countries are increasing medical school enrollment to handle physician shortages. Read the Future Growth section for more information.

4. The capability of influencing future doctors. As the first point of contact for future doctors in their medical field, you are changing lives. This career gives you the capacity to shape and greatly influence the knowledge and skills of future doctors.

5. Medical education is broad-based. Dr. Bec explained that there are multiple aspects of being a medical educator such as research, evaluation, and program design. If one has a good skill set in a particular area, it can be put to good use. If not, the skills needed can be acquired.[93]

Some challenges to becoming a medical educator are:

1. Entry into this career is a challenge. Although some universities train first-time medical educators, most universities rely on their medical educators to recommend qualified colleagues.

2. Academic tenure takes time. Academic tenure (existing in only certain countries) is an indefinite academic appointment post that can only be terminated due to extraordinary circumstances.[99]

Future Growth

A physician shortage in the US and Canada will lead to an urgent call to increase the medical student population by 20-30%. An increase in medical student population will increase the need for medical educators and support staff. This will necessitate evaluation and expansion of existing medical educational programs.[100]

The healthcare landscape is rapidly transforming. In the era of digitalized healthcare systems, medical education must also evolve. We must advance in the areas of virtual reality, augmented reality, and artificial intelligence. As medical technology increases so will the surplus of medical information and knowledge. There is a constant need to select and integrate the most evidence-based and data-driven medical education practices. Furthermore, there is a continuous need to remind individuals of the humanistic aspect of medicine, even regarding medical technologies. Physicians will encounter a growing number of older adults with chronic conditions brought on by prolonged lifespan. Hence, medical educators must evolve as well to ensure that learning is supported across the continuum.[99,100,101]

In the US, the American Medical Association (AMA) launched the Accelerating Change in Medical Education Initiative in 2013 which currently has 37 member schools in its consortium. This project focuses on preparing new doctors for 21st century health care through curricular innovations. It supplies aspiring physicians with the knowledge and experience to navigate digital health technology to address social determinants of health and optimize quality patient care.[101,102]

Now What?

1. Evaluate your skillset. Dr. Bec suggests that individuals take time to reflect on the skill sets they possess and define what they are good at.[93]

2. Get involved with the medical education community. Dr. Bec added:

   > See if there is a local group of educators or a local training organization in your area. Where is your closest university and what opportunities exist there? Start thinking about where the opportunities might be and actively get in touch with people in those areas to express your interest. What inevitably happens is that, when you express interest, they will come and grab you when they need someone.[93]

3. Build a speaking portfolio. Whether it is a small class of ten people or a larger audience of 100 participants, practice speaking and teaching in public. Pick three medical or health topics that you can competently teach. Remember to keep a record of your speaking gigs. This will come in handy when you interview for a medical educator position.

About Dr. Bec

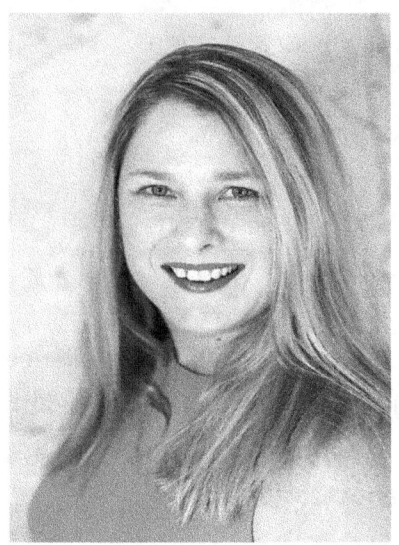

Rebecca Stewart, MBBS, FRACGP, FANZAHPE, FARGP, GCTertEd, MClinEd, PCEval earned her Bachelor of Medicine and Bachelor of Surgery degree from the University of Queensland in Brisbane, Australia in 1996. She completed her Fellowship of the Royal Australian College of General Practitioners (FRACGP) in 2001. She has also completed numerous post graduate courses and qualifications including a Certificate in Women's Health from RACOG in 1999, Graduate Certificate in Tertiary Education (GCTertEd) in 2005, Master of Clinical Education (MClinEd) from Flinders University in 2010, Certificate in Primary Skin Cancer Medicine in 2011, and Certificate in Skin Cancer Therapeutics in 2016.

Dr. Bec also earned her Postgraduate Certificate in Evaluation (PCEval) from Melbourne University in 2015. She completed her Fellowship of the Australia and New Zealand Association of Health Professional Educators (FANZAHHPE) in 2018 and a Fellowship of Advanced Rural General Practice (FARGP) in 2020. Currently, she is National Clinical Lead for Pathways Information Data Systems at the Royal Australian College of General Practitioners (RACGP).

Dr. Bec is also Independent Medical Education Consultant and Director for Medical Education for Experts Pty Ltd. She works as Research Project Manager for GP Training Queensland. She is Training Organization Accreditation Representative, Curriculum Reviewer, and Examiner for the Royal Australian College of General Practitioners (RAGCP). She is Journal Reviewer for the Australian Journal of General Practice (AJGP), Focus on Health Professional Education (FoHPE), and CHECK Magazine. As a clinician, Dr. Bec still works at the Townsville University Hospital as Senior Medical Officer in the Cardiac Clinics Department.

In her free time, she runs, cycles, paddleboards, and kayaks. She enjoys gourmet cooking, embroidery, felting, and dressmaking. She also dabbles in instructional and web design. Dr. Bec loves watching sports with her husband and two daughters, particularly rugby and cricket. She enjoys exploring the vast expanse of Australia.

Chapter 13

Medical Reviewer

Overview

Job Title	Medical Reviewer / Clinical Reviewer
Salary Range	Average annual income in the US: $71,298. Ranges from $36,500 (25th percentile) to $93,000 (75th percentile)[103]
Education	Knowledge of medical terminology, government, and insurance guidelines required
Training	On-the-job training available in some companies
Skills/Talents	Compassionate, humble, focused, detail-oriented
Sample Companies	Advanced Medical Reviews, AllMed Healthcare Management Inc, Alicare Medical Management, BHM Healthcare Solutions, Cigna, Claims Eval Inc, Concentra, EviCore, ExamWorks, Health Claim Review, Healthcare Quality Strategies Inc, Independent Medical Expert Consulting Services, Kepro Physician Reviewers, MedConnect VA, Managed Medical Review Organization, MES Solutions, MLS Group of Companies, MSLA, Nexus Medical, Physicians' Review Network, Prest & Associates, Network Medical Review, R3 Continuum, Reliable Review Services[104]
Projected Job Growth	Approximately 11% increase in the US from 2018-2028[105]

What is a Medical Reviewer?

A medical reviewer reviews and examines medical documents for accuracy, completion, and correlation with an insurance or legal claim. Medical reviewers work closely with hospitals, clinics, insurance companies, government agencies, and independent auditing firms. They review and audit all medical documentation in hospitals and clinics that maybe vital to a hospital's accreditation or an insurance company's reimbursement. They also coordinate meetings with medical staff to check physician notes for completion and proficiency. They report any evidence of neglect or haphazard submission for compliance and corrections.[103]

Sample Case

Dr. Luis Asensio earned his Doctor of Medicine degree from the Universidad Central del Este, Dominican Republic in 2008. He currently works as Lead Medical Reviewer for MedConnectVa in Tampa, Florida. Dr. Luis stated:

> I realized it was time to change my career when I decided to move to the United States. I had a period of my life where I worked as a clinician but, suddenly, it was time to consider other positions. It is a sensitive and personal journey. I came here to the United States because my wife was diagnosed with a heart condition – a very rare heart condition – that could not be treated where we were at. When she was diagnosed with it, she was pregnant. So, we had an aggravating factor there. At the time, I had all my papers ready to come here to the States. I was a legal resident, and I could work as a legal resident. My first goal was to have medical insurance and, of course, I was leaning toward careers that relate to my background. Fortunately – I believe it was a blessing from God – I landed with a company as a medical reviewer for the Veterans Administration (VA). Eventually, that led me on a path of understanding VA idiosyncrasies.
>
> Within my independent auditing firm, I act as a link between veterans and the attorneys defending them for a claimed condition that either started in service or was due to service. I work with doctors and medical experts in charge of assessing the claimed condition in accordance with the veteran's benefits. We discuss every conceivable angle to support the veteran. I work as an intermediary between these two positions. I am similar to a translator from the legal language to the medical language.[106]

Roles and Responsibilities

Some medical reviewers work for clinics or providers. They receive a list of patients to audit from insurance companies. Often, insurance companies are looking for confirmation of assessment of a chronic condition. For instance, suppose the insurance company receives a reimbursement claim from a specialist that Jane Doe was diagnosed with diabetes with neurological symptoms. The insurance company will seek to confirm this assessment with Jane's primary care physician. They notify the primary care physician to audit Jane Doe's charts for diabetes with neurological symptoms. The medical reviewer for that clinic will check Jane's charts from the current year's visits for medical codes for diabetes with neurological symptoms. If the medical codes are present, the medical reviewer communicates with the insurance through supplementary documentation or portal and confirms the chronic condition. If the medical codes are not current, the medical reviewer will speak with the primary care physician to assess a possible additional diagnosis for the upcoming visit.

Other medical reviewers work for insurance companies. They receive requests for coverage from doctors' clinics for medical services, procedures, and diagnostics. They check the medical documentation for appropriate criteria, gather more information if necessary, and perform a detailed audit. Then, they analyze and communicate the approval or disapproval of the medical service, procedure, or diagnostic to the doctor's clinic.

Still other medical reviewers work for independent auditing firms hired by attorneys or other third parties. A typical day in Dr. Luis' independent auditing firm consists of receiving documentation regarding veteran patients with special consideration to client privacy. The medical documents contain patients' health records before, during, and after service. The medical information can range from five pages to as many as 300-400 pages. He assesses the medical history to connect a claimed condition to an event in active military service such as trauma, chemical exposure, or work-related health issues. Utilizing his medical background, Dr. Luis reviews the story and assesses, from a medical perspective, whether there is a possible connection to the veteran's condition and his time in service. He then communicates to legal representatives and medical experts the best approach to satisfy specific guidelines for connecting a veteran's claimed condition to service.[106]

Skills, Education, Certification, and Training

There is no formal education or training necessary to join this field. However, organizations generally look for individuals with experience in medical terminology, government, and insurance guidelines. However, a handful of healthcare organizations are willing to invest in training newcomers in this field.

Dr. Luis credits his background as an international medical graduate and on-the-job company training for preparing him to be a medical reviewer. To be exemplary in a medical reviewer position, Dr. Luis believes compassion is the number one strength needed to succeed. He stated:

> You are dealing with military veterans with very touching and sensitive stories. I see a person with a story behind the condition. I think compassion is the engine that makes you excel in this type of job. It makes a difference because you are dealing with people who have struggled and gone through a lot. You need humbleness and should come with an open mind to learn because you deal with attorneys and medical experts who will reshape your perspectives. Humility allows you to listen to others. Thirdly, you have to be detail-oriented. You will sift through a lot of documentation and must view every piece of information as something potentially relevant.
>
> I was very blessed that my first company in the United States trained me to completely understand the veteran community and the Veterans Administration system.[106]

Pros and Cons:

Some advantages to becoming a medical reviewer are:

1. You can work remotely. This is another career where you need a laptop and secure Wi-Fi access. Most of your documents will be in the company's system, so there is no need for a physical office space. You will be dealing with confidential patient medical records, so most companies have an added cybersecurity layer for logins and authentications.

2. Your hours are flexible. Companies generally expect a 9 a.m. to 5 p.m. workday to complete assignments. But, as long as you log eight hours, you can extend your day to 7 p.m. or 8 p.m. and utilize your mornings for a doctor's appointment or luncheon. Flexibility is essential for those with younger families who may need to take a child to daycare or school.

3. You work with different personalities. A successful future in this career is dependent on making healthy relationships. As a medical reviewer, you will engage with lawyers and doctors constantly. As an IMG, you already possess many of the skills required to relate with colleagues in this field.

4. You indirectly improve someone's quality of life. Dr. Luis reported:

> Sometimes you don't hear from a veteran for months after you completed their case. Then, you receive an email thanking you and the company for your work telling you that it has changed their life. It makes my day knowing that all the effort and hours invested to untangle the medical aspects of a case was worth it.[106]

Some challenges to becoming a medical reviewer are:

1. Finding the first company to train you is daunting. Most companies require medical reviewer experience. As a newcomer, it is hard to find that one company that is willing to invest in training and teaching you the ins and outs of the industry.

2. You will do a lot of reading. Your company will assign you cases where you must thoroughly read all medical records and supporting documents. It is essential not to skim through the details because a phrase can make or break your case.

Future Growth

There will be an approximately 11% increase in the US from 2018 to 2028.[105] The upward surge in the medical review industry is partly due to increasing medical malpractice costs and payouts.[107,108,109] The presence of stricter guidelines helps alleviate malpractice costs and boost medical review procedures to improve patient care, safety, and quality.

Now What?

1. Research availabilities with the sample companies (MedConnect VA, MSLA, MLS Group of Companies, Prest & Associates, Network Medical Review, Kepro, ExamWorks, R3 Continuum, Physicians' Review Network, Prium, Genex Services, Managed Medical Review Organization, MES Solutions, Advanced Medical Reviews, Reliable Review Services, Concentra, EviCore, Nexus Medical, HQSI, QTC, Cigna, BHM Healthcare Solutions, Maximus, Independent Medical Expert Consulting Services).[104] Read through their requirements and assess your compatibility.

2. Leverage LinkedIn. Network with someone from your prospective organization. Search for the company name in the search bar, and filter by the "People" icon. This will give you a comprehensive list of possible connections. Send a "Connect" invite and always "Add a Note." The "Add a Note" section is a free tool on LinkedIn. Write a short paragraph on why you are reaching out. Here is an example:

   > Hello Sir/Madam,
   >
   > I am looking to expand my connection in the field of medical review. I saw that you work for XYZ organization. I would love to connect, hear about your experiences, and gain advice on how to leverage my medical degree for this career. Can we do a virtual coffee?
   >
   > Sincerely,
   > Your name

   Set up a Zoom virtual coffee. Your goal is to give your time to get their time. Hear their story. Then share your story and what you are looking for. Genuinely get to know the person. Keep in touch with them every month. You will create a lasting impression and be first on their call list when there are future openings within their organization.

3. Apply to the position advertised.

   When asked for his last piece of advice, Dr. Luis advised:

   > Do not underestimate your knowledge. There are many opportunities out there. I landed in something that I never would have thought I would be doing, but deeply love. This career relates to what I did in the Dominican Republic. It prepared me. When I came here, I hoped to find something related to medicine that would utilize my medical knowledge. So, do not underestimate your knowledge and your preparation. There are companies seeking individuals with your knowledge and your preparation. I would encourage every international medical graduate to not give up. There is something out there for you.[106]

About Dr. Luis

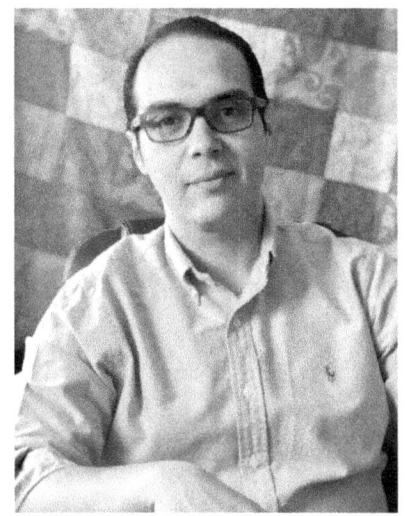

Dr. Luis Asensio earned his Doctor of Medicine degree from the Universidad Central del Este, Dominican Republic in 2008. In addition to being a practitioner, he worked as Clinical Documentation Auditor for Clinical Del Nino, San Pedro de Macorís, Dominican Republic from 2009-2012. He was promoted to Medical Manager and, later, to Clinical Documentation Audit Department Director for the same multi-specialty clinical facility from 2012-2017. He developed clinical and surgical treatment guidelines and oversaw the in-hospital practice of more than 50 medical providers. During that time, he was also a Christian minister and pastor of a small local church. In 2016, his wife was diagnosed with a rare cardiac condition while pregnant with their second son. Without thinking twice, Luis left his career and ministry behind to pursue treatment for his wife in the United States. In 2017, he became Medical Reviewer for VA-related clinical examinations for MSLA, a United Health Group. In 2018, he became Lead Medical Reviewer for MedConnectVa, a fast-growing company that provides high-quality medical opinions for veterans.

Currently, Dr. Luis' wife and two kids are well and they all live in Tampa Bay, Florida.

Chapter 14

Medical Science Liaison

Overview

Job Title	Medical Science Liaison (MSL) / Medical Liaison / Medical Science Manager / Scientific Manager / Clinical Liaison
Salary Range	Average annual income in the US: $169,541. Varies by region, industry type, education, and experience[110]
Education	Doctorate degree (MD, PharmD, PhD)
Training	MSL Board Certification (MSL-BC), clinical, research, or scientific field experience[111]
Skills/Talents	Written and verbal communication skills, excellent interpersonal skills, analytical skills, adaptability, flexibility, clinical trial design, pharmacogenomics, evidence-based medicine skills
Sample Companies	AbbVie, Agenus, Baxter, Bluebird Bio, Blueprint Medicines, Eli Lilly, Eurofins, Hoffmann-La Roche, Kala Pharmaceuticals, Incyte Corporation, Intercept Pharmaceuticals Inc, IPSEN, Sage Therapeutics, Seattle Genetics, Servier Pharmaceuticals, Syneos Health, The Medical Affairs Company, ViiV Healthcare,
Projected Job Growth	Approximately 7% increase in the US from 2018-2028[110]

What is a Medical Science Liaison?

Medical science liaisons (MSLs) were primarily established by Upjohn Pharmaceuticals in 1967.[110] They are scientific professionals who act as bridges between healthcare companies and physicians. They are assigned geographic areas and regions that require extensive travel, accounting for 60-80% of their time on the job. They are generally employed under the Medical Affairs departments of pharmaceutical, medical device, biotechnology, managed care, and other healthcare companies.[110,112] They specialize in various therapeutic areas (cardiology, CNS, hematology, oncology, etc.) and disease states (cardiovascular disease, diabetes, etc.). They are responsible for creating a connection between healthcare companies and medical doctors, hospitals, and decision makers.[111,113]

Sample Case

Dr. Carlos Madrigal-Iberri earned his Doctor of Medicine degree from Universidad Autonoma de Coahuila Facultad de Medicina Unidad Saltillo, Coahuila, Mexico in 2013. He pivoted to a nontraditional career and became a medical science liaison. He spent his last year in medicine at the University of Illinois Medical Center at Chicago in a Cardiology Clinical Experience rotation. Dr. Carlos stated:

> I realized there are a lot of different ways you can perform medicine beyond being a specialist. When I completed my studies, I applied for residency with a lot of doubts as to my medical specialization of surgery. It was difficult to challenge the pressure I received from peers, parents, and friends. I went for six, maybe eight, months in my surgery residency when I was offered a job in a pharmaceutical company as their medical science liaison. They offered me three times the money I was making as a resident. So, I decided to try it for a year. That was in 2017.[114]

Roles and Responsibilities

MSLs are vital ingredients in building rapport with key opinion leaders and decision-makers within their organization. They are responsible for engaging internal stakeholders in healthcare companies by serving as subject-matter experts. They provide training and support for clinical, marketing, product development, and sales teams.[113] They also represent their healthcare company in medical conferences and engage in meetings where they deliver complex information.[110] Dr. Carlos stated that MSLs have a lot of meetings within the company to align strategies. Also, he has an upcoming Medical Congress where he needs to train the speaker to present all the relevant science surrounding the disease.[114]

MSLs create transparency from healthcare organizations to the medical community. MSLs are responsible for collaborating with external stakeholders in the medical community and regulatory agencies by sharing insights, communicating scientific data, supporting external research activities, and developing engagement plans and programs to improve health outcomes.[110,113] They also analyze scientific trends and clinical practices by monitoring clinical literature for new developments. They help ensure effective use of products by providing advice on treatment advancements and input on relevant clinical data.[111,112] One of Dr. Carlos' projects included round table discussions with key opinion leaders in Mexico to create a national technique to treat heart failure. Dr. Carlos stated:

> We are responsible for communicating scientific development of clinical trials and improving communication systems between stakeholders. You align messages on innovative therapies. You discuss new scientific papers.
>
> MSLs become peers of physicians in clinics and hospitals. We provide continuous medical education to other physicians. We also educate nurses because they play such an important role in patient outcomes.[114]

Skills, Education, Certification, and Training

Often, healthcare companies seek MSLs with extensive knowledge on epidemiology, pharmacy, medicine, health economics, and health policy. Most prospective MSLs have a doctorate in life sciences, doctor of medicine (MD), doctor of pharmacy (PharmD), or doctor of philosophy (PhD) with extensive experience in a specific therapeutic specialization.[115] In fact, a 2020 survey of 2,034 MSL professionals from 67 countries showed that 85% in the US and 77% globally hold a doctorate degree.[113]

The Medical Science Liaison Society (MSL Society) is a nonprofit organization that is exclusively dedicated to advancing the growth and development of the international MSL profession. They provide tools and resources for prospective and established MSL professionals. The MSL Society has recently developed a professional certification called the MSL Board Certification (MSL-BC) to set industry standards for the MSL profession.[113]

To become a successful MSL, excellent written and verbal communication skills are needed. Dr. Carlos stated:

It is essential to improve networking opportunities with professionals and people you work with every day. As an MSL, you are on a transformative journey to becoming a better leader. One must learn to be grounded in communication, learning how to present data correctly and how to analyze databases. You must also have passion for what you do and a deep commitment to science. As an MSL, you will be an active, lifelong learner as you teach, educate, and reveal the science behind everything.[114]

Pros and Cons

Some advantages to becoming a medical science liaison are:

1. Excellent financial compensation. This profession's entry-level position starts at $138,000 and averages close to $160,000. The income increases as you gain experience.[110,116]

2. There is extensive traveling. Pre-COVID-19, this profession traveled 60%-80% of the time. You will be assigned a geographical territory to cover. You will be required to attend multiple conferences a year. It is not unusual to participate in two conferences in one week in different regions of the country.

3. There are unique opportunities to network. You will jump from one meeting to another, from one conference to another. Your ability to network will be tremendously tested. You will engage with thought leaders in the industry. Therefore, being able to hold a scientific conversation with ease is a significant advantage.

Some challenges to becoming a medical science liaison are:

1. This an extremely competitive market and one of the top ten best alternatives for PhDs who wish to transition from the academic or laboratory field. Dr. Carlos advised:

    > This is a competitive role. Be sure that you want to pursue this career. Knock on as many doors as you can and go for it. Be an agent of change. Just like being a physician, many people will hear your voice. Make it loud. Make it clear. Let us do our best to improve the world together.[114]

2. There is extensive traveling. This can be a pro or a con, depending on your preferences and lifestyle. This may not be a feasible alternative for someone with a young family.

Future Growth

The MSL profession has grown tremendously over the last 30 years. From 2018 to 2028, there is a projected job growth of approximately 7% in the US.[110] From 2020 onward, there is an estimated growth of 20% to 35% in South America and Asia, respectively.[115]

The MSL profession grows with the complexity of medicine. With the increasing shift toward cutting edge therapies, medicine grows more complex and molecular. With the increase in emphasis on rare diseases, the therapeutic management of complex drugs and action mechanisms becomes more complicated.[115]

Now What?

1. Take advantage of scientific conferences in your therapeutic specialty. Try networking with sales representatives from the vendor booths. Be genuinely interested in their products. For example, you might have an off-label question. Ask the sales representative if there is a medical colleague present to provide you with an answer.[117]

2. Network with MSLs in your therapeutic and geographic area. Try LinkedIn again. Search for "Medical Science Liaison" in the search bar, then click on the "People" Icon to narrow it down to MSL professionals. Send them a "Connect" invite with an "Add a Note." Be genuine, say something such as:

   > Dear Sir/Madam,
   >
   > I am interested in transitioning to the MSL world. I would love to hear about your story and your experiences and gain some advice on how to leverage my medical degree for this career. Can we set up a virtual coffee this week?
   >
   > Sincerely,
   > Your name

During your Zoom virtual coffee, you can ask about their career experience, including their journey to becoming an MSL, what they currently do, and what they foresee doing in the future. Genuinely get to know the person. Keep in touch with them every month. You never know when you will need to contact this person in the future. You will create a lasting impression and be first on their call list when there are future openings within their organization.

3. Read *How to Break into Your First MSL Role* by Dr. Samuel Dyer. Dr. Dyer is a hiring manager who details how to search, apply for, and interview for an MSL position.[117]

About Dr. Carlos

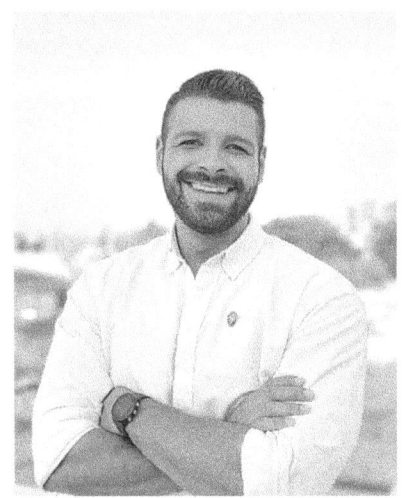

Dr. Carlos Madrigal-Iberri earned his Doctor of Medicine degree from Universidad Autonoma de Coahuila Facultad de Medicina Unidad Saltillo, Coahuila, Mexico in 2013. He completed a Cardiology Clinical Experience and worked as Lab Assistant in the Physiology and Biophysics Department at the University of Illinois, Chicago in 2013. He was Clinical Research Coordinator and Sub Investigator in HIV/AIDS at the Infectious Diseases and Immunology Clinic of the Instituto Nacional de Ciencias Medicas y Nutrition "Salvador Zubiran" from 2015-2017. He completed a Diploma in Diabetes certified by Universidad La Salle and Sociedad Mexicana de Nutricion y Endocrinologia in 2017 and a Diploma in Experimental Clinical Research in Health certified by Universidad Nacional Autonoma de Mexico in 2018. He worked as an E-Medical Science Liaison in Metabolism at Janssen Pharmaceuticals from 2017-2018.

Dr. Carlos also completed a Diploma in Pharmacoeconomics certified by Universidad La Salle in 2018 and Diploma in Management Skills and High-Performance Teams certified by Universidad del Valle de Mexico in 2019. Since 2018 he has been employed as Medical Science Liaison in Cardiovascular and Metabolism at Novartis Pharmaceuticals.

Dr. Carlos is passionate about One Young World, an international leadership organization for young people. He defines himself as a social activist who enjoys helping young leaders achieve goals outlined in the Sustainable Development Goals 2030 developed by the United Nations General Assembly. He is committed to leaving a better world behind. His other interests include CrossFit, watching TV series and movies, reading, cooking, and playing with his dog, Mila.

Chapter 15

Medical Scientist

Overview

Job Title	Medical Scientist / Researcher / Research Scientist
Salary Range	Annual average income in the US: $88,790. Ranges from $50,000 (10th percentile) to $120,000 (90th percentile)[118]
Education and Training	PhD or MD. Most companies require research experience
Skills/Talents	Project management skills, problem-solving and analytical skills, technical writing, critical thinking, written and verbal communication skills
Sample companies	Johnson & Johnson, Pfizer Inc, Pharmaceutical Product Development (PPD) Inc, Thermo Fisher Scientific Inc
Projected Job Growth	Approximately 6% increase in the US from 2019-2029[118]

What is a Medical Scientist?

A medical scientist conducts research to improve overall human health. They are responsible for collecting, organizing, and analyzing data to find a solution to a disease entity or condition. They work in pharmaceuticals, universities, governmental public health agencies, and medical device companies.

Sample Case

Numan Majeed, MBBS, MPhil, (FCPS) earned his Bachelor of Medicine and Bachelor of Surgery degree from Muhammad Medical College in Mirpur Khas, Pakistan. Currently, he maintains his medical practice as a pathologist and works as a medical scientist. Dr. Numan stated:

> I began my research journey the second year of medical school. I was active with the Asian Medical Students' Association – International (AMSA-International). It was at that point where I got the idea of doing research. I realized I wanted to conduct research and mentor others as well. I decided I could augment my pathology work with research as an alternative pathway. Currently, I do my own research and conduct research workshops, conferences, and training for undergraduates and graduates about research techniques.[119]

Roles and Responsibilities

Medical scientists start with aligning their research objectives with organizational goals. They design medical studies and clinical trials with the goal of finding solutions to medical conditions and illnesses. They set project goals and create plans of action. They formulate efficient research processes and facilitate research assignments. For example, some medical scientists oversee the development phases of a drug or medical device. They then utilize various methodologies and resources to obtain the most recent and relevant data. They perform fieldwork, experiments, interviews, clinical trials, and concept tests on the sample population.

Next is data interpretation. Medical scientists compound, integrate, and analyze their findings. They look for correlations, causations, and connections between health conditions and risk factors. Some use software for data analytics, which also involves checking for errors and inconsistencies. They compile and organize their findings in charts, graphs, and diagrams, followed by reporting and presenting these findings to management and clients.

Research projects vary depending on the industry. Dr. Numan has worked with public health issues. He explored use of the internet among medical students in comparison with eating habits and other addictive habits.[119] He also examined Cystatin-C, developing a predictive model which used biochemical markers for gestational diabetes. Dr. Numan stated:

We previously used fundoscopy for diagnosis which is subjectively dependent on the opinion of the ophthalmologist. I proposed using biomarkers for diagnosis and staging of the disease rather than fundoscopy, which has ambiguities.[119]

Dr. Numan's other published research projects include *Comparison of Procalcitonin and Hematological Ratios in Cord Blood as Early Predictive Marker of Neonatal Sepsis*[120]; *Association of Liver Function Derangements with Disease Severity in COVID-19 Patients*[121]; and *Comparison of three different bone graft methods for single segment lumbar tuberculosis: A retrospective single-center cohort study*[122] among many others. The imagination is the limit for any research project.

Skills, Education, Certification, and Training

To become a medical scientist, you must have an underlying passion for systemic investigation. An MD/DO degree is a great asset because many medical universities require research for graduation. Other medical doctors attain advanced degrees. For example, an epidemiologist might complete a Master of Public Health degree, a biochemist/biophysicist may complete a PhD in Biochemistry or Biophysics, and a geneticist may complete a PhD in Genetics. Furthermore, if you want to work with clinical trials, a Clinical Research Certification will boost your application. Dr. Numan stated:

> I am an example of someone who is self-taught. When you are starting up, all you need to do is read, read, read. As in medical school, you learn by reading your textbooks. It is important to learn from all the available knowledge and information. It is essential to learn as much as you can from all the different materials out there.[119]

Pros and Cons

Some advantages to becoming a medical scientist are:

1. You always work in teams. You will collaborate with various departments from the initiation until the completion of your research projects. For pharmaceutical and medical device companies, you work closely with the Quality Assurance and Regulatory department to conduct risk assessments.

2. You are part of a close-knit community. You will be a guide for other scientists. Dr. Numan stated:

> My colleagues come to me for advice. I am encouraged that I am helping people. For me, a great incentive is when people senior to me from my institute, and other institutes, ask for my advice. For example, during my master's program, I had a senior who was working on his PhD program project who came to me for guidance.[119]

3. Your research experience from medical school will come in handy. Most medical schools have research requirements for graduation. From this, you learned to identify a problem, create a hypothesis, test the idea through robust methodology, collect samples, analyze your selections, and write a conclusion.

4. Your research work may be used as a guideline in medicine. Dr. Numan explained that guidelines are always being updated. He stated:

   > Scientists conduct research and publish articles. Those articles are then used to make guidelines. Knowledge is power. To be a facilitator of expertise, primarily in the field of medicine, is such an essential aspect of the career.[119]

Some challenges to becoming a medical scientist are:

1. You will need experience to join this field. This is not an entry-level career. You will need experience in conducting research and producing publications to begin work in this field. If you want to work with pharmaceutical companies, you will need to show that you understand laboratory procedures and processes.

2. Some organizations may offer temporary positions. If you want to work with government agencies or research institutions, your job may be limited to a certain timeframe. The timeframe generally has an expiration secondary to its grant funding. Be mindful when applying for these positions.

3. You need to publish or perish. This cliché in the research community is generally true for government and research institutions. Your research aims are to publish your outcomes, especially if you plan on sustaining grant funding from the government or private sector.

Future Growth

Employment for medical scientists is expected to grow by approximately 6% in the US from 2019-2029.[118] The demand for medical scientists has increased due to the aging population living longer, increased chronic condition rates, and increased pharmaceutical resilience. Medical scientists are needed for research advancements in Alzheimer's diseases, HIV/AIDS, cancer, and other chronic conditions.

Now What?

1. Leverage your research work. Dust off those thesis papers or case studies from medical school. If they were not published, and the timeframe is still feasible, try submitting your article to peer-reviewed journals. You have already done the majority of the work. This is a perfect time to get recognized for the work you have already completed.

2. Join a journal as a peer-reviewer. Use Google search or other search engines for a journal of interest. Check the credentials needed to join as a peer-reviewer. Apply to a handful of journals. This will add to your credibility as an expert in the field.

3. Network. Find a connection. LinkedIn is your best friend. Search for a "Medical Scientist" in your area and "Connect." When sending that invitation for a connection, "Add a note." Express your interest in why you are reaching out to this individual. Be keen to learn about their story. Share your story and aspirations. Your message should look something like this:

> Hello Sir/Madam,
>
> I am looking to expand my connection in the field of medical research. I saw that you work for XYZ organization. I would love to connect, hear about your experiences, and gain advice on how to leverage my medical degree for this career. Can we do a virtual coffee?
>
> Sincerely,
> Your name

Set up a Zoom virtual coffee. Your goal is to give your time to get their time. Hear their story. Then share your story and what you are looking for. Genuinely get to know the person.

Keep in touch with them every month. You will create a lasting impression and be first on their call list when there are future openings within their organization.

4. Apply for jobs. Now that you have done the hard work, it is time to test the waters and apply for a job as a medical scientist. Take the time to read job descriptions in their entirety. Tailor your resume or CV to contain wording from the job description. Write a stellar cover letter. Show them how amazing you are. Highlight your analytical, writing, and problem-solving skills.

About Dr. Numan

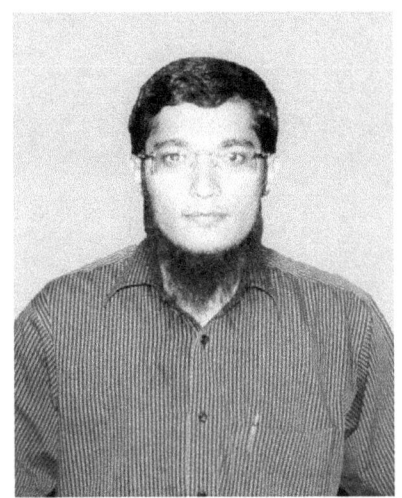

Numan Mejeed, MBBS, MPhil, (FCPS) earned his Bachelor of Medicine and Bachelor of Surgery degree from Muhammad Medical College and his Master of Philosophy degree in Army Medical College in Mirpur Khas, Pakistan. Besides working as Chemical Pathologist and Lecturer for Army Medical College National University of Medical Sciences, he also worked as Research Associate for Public Health and Research in Lahore, Pakistan. He was also Research Associate for the Department of Genetics (Developmental Genetics Lab) in 2014 and Research Assistant for the Department of Cell Biology (Cardiovascular and Xenotransplant Lab) in 2013 at King Faisal Specialist Hospital and Research Center, Riyadh, Saudi Arabia.

Dr. Numan has 47 publications (27 journal publications [9ISI Impact, 10 PubMed], and 20 conference presentations). He has also reviewed for several journals including the British Medical Journal, International Journal of Surgery, The Lancet Students Journal, International Journal of Medical Informatics, Journal of Clinical and Diagnostic Research, and Journal of Medical Systems. He served as Editor-in-Chief for the Journal of Asian Medical Students.

Chapter 16

Pharmaceutical Ethics and Compliance Continuum

Overview

Job Title	Ethics and Compliance Associate / Ethics and Compliance Manager / Ethics and Compliance Director / Vice President of Ethics and Compliance / Chief Ethics and Compliance Officer (titles depend on companies and local practices)
Salary Range	Ethics and Compliance Officer average annual income in the US: $157,350. Ranges from $100,189 (10th percentile) to $222,668 (90th percentile). Incomes vary by region, education, certifications, and number of years of experience[123]
Education	Most companies prefer a robust educational background in risk management, compliance, finance, accounting, policy, or law
Training	On-the-job training available. Prior managerial experience is recommended for roles with people management. Prior experience with local and state government laws and regulations is recommended
Skills/Talents	Risk management and analytical skills, verbal and written communication skills, managerial skills
Sample companies	AbbVie Inc, Bayer AG, Eli Lilly, GlaxoSmithKline Plc, GSK, Hoffman-La Roche Ltd, Intercept Pharmaceuticals, Johnson & Johnson, Merck & Co Inc, Novartis, Pfizer, Sanofi, Syneos Health, Takeda
Projected Job Growth	See the Future Growth section for trends in the industry

What is a Pharmaceutical Ethics and Compliance Continuum?

An essential factor of pharmaceutical corporate responsibility is the overarching purpose of the ethics and compliance program to prevent corruption and protect human lives. The compliance program is led by commercial corporate leadership and its purpose is to promote a culture of the highest ethical standards within the company. Positions in the pharmaceutical ethics and compliance continuum are mainly non-clinical – administrative, supervisory, and executive in nature – and include pharmaceutical ethics and compliance associate, manager, vice president of ethics and compliance, and chief ethics and compliance officer. These positions will be discussed in more detail later in the chapter.

Sample Case

Dr. Swee Kheng Khor earned his Doctor of Medicine degree from the National University of Malaysia. His story is one of resilience as he pivoted from traditional medicine to pharmaceutical medical affairs to pharmaceutical ethics and compliance. His current venture is in public health, health policies, and health systems. Dr. SK stated:

> It is worth mentioning that my journey took 15-16 years, so it was not an overnight story. My father wanted me to practice medicine, and I thought it was a very good choice for a young person who did not know what he wanted to do at the age of 19-20 years old. Upon graduation, I started working as a doctor in Malaysia. I spent four and a half years in the Malaysian government working for the Malaysian Ministry of Health as a doctor. I then looked for something a little bit more holistic, perhaps at the intersection between science and the arts to have a greater impact.[124]

Dr. SK made plans to transition away from traditional medicine. He prepared a safety net by maintaining his internal medicine practice before he explored alternative careers. He stated:

> I found that another strategy for pivoting to another career was having a little bit of an idea of where I want to go. So, I joined the American pharmaceutical industry which was one of the larger ones in the world. I spent nine years doing two main things for them. First, I worked in medical affairs, scientific governance, scientific education, and clinical research which were based in Singapore. Later, the company spun off into two companies. I went with the new company, and there was an opportunity to be based in Dubai working

in ethics and compliance. I was lucky to find a mentor who was willing to take a chance on me as someone who did not have compliance experience in the Middle East or Africa. I spent four and a half years in Dubai and was sent to Shanghai on a short-term assignment, before being promoted to lead the compliance team for Eastern Europe, Russia and the CIS countries, the Middle East, and Africa.[124]

Roles and Responsibilities

Ethics and compliance managers or analysts oversee the daily operations of the company's ethics and compliance functions, while more senior compliance officers oversee the program's overall direction. They work in pharmaceutical, medical device, and medical insurance companies. This chapter will discuss this career continuum in pharmaceutical companies.

Ethics and compliance manager and director positions have three components: creating policies consistent with local laws and standards, training and educating employees on these policies, and monitoring compliance with policies. Primarily, these professionals create policies that meet and follow company protocols, industry standards, and federal laws where the company operates. Company policies include a code of ethics, anti-bribery and anti-corruption laws, professional practices, risk management, mitigating third-party risks, professional practices, and upholding human rights. Industry regulatory standards vary by country and by region.[125]

Secondly, managers and directors train staff and communicate policies. Compliance managers and directors must effectively ensure understanding and follow through with policies and regulations. They persuade and influence the why and how of compliance. Dr. SK said:

> It is not enough to say, 'I've trained them.' People may say, 'I don't understand,' or they may not be persuaded. Encourage, inspire, motivate, and use the tools necessary to get people to comply.[124]

Lastly, managers and directors monitor compliance. They ensure adherence to all protocols and legislation that govern the development and use of medications. If deviations are found, they prevent, investigate, and remediate violations of regulations, laws, and policies. Dr. SK went on to state:

> The best medicines should always be prescribed independently by doctors, and purchasing decisions made independently by payers or insurers. Also, health economists and health systems specialists should never be at the mercy of any

form of corruption or bribery. The compliance program ensures that the way we market our products, conduct ourselves, and interact with health professionals and government officials are transparent and conducted in an ethical manner.[124]

Skills, Education, Certification, and Training

To get into the pharmaceutical ethics and compliance field, you may need to start as an analyst or manager. Dr. SK recalled his experience:

> There are no university degrees to be a compliance officer, so you must be open to listening and receiving advice, counsel, and wisdom from people who have gone before you. There is a lot that you can learn. Secondly, there is a high and very steep learning curve, and that learning curve requires a lot of reading. Listening to people is one thing; reading is another. You cannot rely solely on people for every source of information.
>
> Traditionally, people who are compliance officers are accountants or lawyers. Well, I am a physician and I brought different skill sets. When your company wants to run particular patient support programs, you must understand the purpose of those programs and how they affect doctors and patients.[124]

To become a successful manager or director in this field, you need to show a strong knowledge base for risk management, compliance, policy, and law. Most companies require additional educational background and industry certifications. Dr. SK agreed:

> To move from one career to another, often you will need an education that will help you re-label yourself and give you new skill sets.[124]

Pros and Cons

Some advantages of a career in pharmaceutical ethics and compliance are:

1. Great financial compensation. This career provides comfortable monetary compensation and benefits from well-known, well-established companies. The entry-level annual salary is approximately $80,000-$90,000 with increased compensation as you gain more exposure and experience.[123]

2. Good job security. With the technology tsunami, there will be more ethical and compliance policy and regulation changes across all industries, especially pharmaceutical companies. These opportunities will create and sustain adequate job security for this career.

3. Working with leaders. You will coordinate programs with thought leaders internally and externally. You will advocate for policy changes to convince critical stakeholders. Your work will significantly impact the product and services of the company.

Some challenges of a career in pharmaceutical ethics and compliance are:

1. Steep learning curve. This is a foreign industry for most healthcare professionals. To show your determination and passion for this career, it is essential to gain additional knowledge. Taking courses, even a master's program, would boost your candidacy and increase your chances of landing a position.

2. Relocation to another country. Moving to another country may be necessary for some in this career field. Dr. SK said of his time in the industry:

> It is a big adjustment because it is a culture shock. You move from the government sector into the private sector. You move from one country to another country. There is a lot of personal adjustment to new careers, new countries, new industries, and new organizations. The cultural and psychological adaptations are often tougher than the usual professional adaptation.[124]

3. Avid reader and learner. A nimble and flexible attitude is a must. Regulations and laws are frequently changing, so it is essential to be abreast of changes. This will require constant reading and learning from various articles, websites, and industry platforms. Your daily responsibilities will alter based on new and updated developments.

4. Resilience. A resilient individual will move faster in this career continuum. When you begin this career, it may seem unfamiliar. Dr. SK stated:

> You are a newbie in a field with great depth. Therefore, you must work hard and be prepared to get your hands dirty. Be willing to gain the experience needed to adapt well professionally.[124]

Future Growth

The COVID-19 pandemic compelled many companies to operate remotely. This work-from-home trend has ambiguous effects on productivity, ethics, and compliance. Work-from-home employees are more susceptible to stress, anxiety, and isolation, leading to an increased likelihood of cutting corners, bending rules, and making poor decisions.[126]

Companies often own substantial intellectual property such as trademarks, copyrights, patents, and trade secrets that are susceptible to internal theft. Work-from-home employees with access to sensitive information can lead to data leaks. Individuals can become enticed to take pictures of designs or products and sell them to competitors.[126] Hence, the ethics and compliance committee's vigilant monitoring and enforcement of policies is vital to the business.

Also, the US federal government issued essential documents in 2019: the Evaluation of Corporate Compliance Programs from Department of Justice's Criminal and Antitrust Divisions and the Sanctions Compliance Guidance from the Department of Treasury's Office of Foreign Assets. These documents aim to support corporate ethics and compliance programs by crediting a company's efforts and minimizing damages if they suffer losses from compliance issues under US Sentencing Guidelines.[127]

Now What?

1. The primary consideration is how much education you need to move forward. Before jumping into a master's degree, try online courses in ethics, compliance, policy, or law. This is an excellent avenue to find out if this field is something you want to invest time and money in. Try Edx, Udemy, or Coursera. Udemy courses cost an average of $12.99 on their sale dates, while Coursera ranges from free to $300, depending on whether or not you want a signed certificate of completion. Edx is another option you can try.

2. If you determine this is the career for you, it is time to complete a certification program or Master of Health Economics, Policy, and Law degree. There are some certifications offered from Edx or Coursera websites as a cheaper, yet functional, alternative. If you want to go the route of earning a master's degree, bear in mind that there are international institutions that have prestigious programs. Some even offer scholarships to prospective students.

3. Network with someone from your prospective organization. The best resource is LinkedIn. Search for the company name in the search bar, and filter by the "People" icon. This will

give you a comprehensive list of possible connections. Send a "Connect" invite and always "Add a Note." The "Add a Note" section is a free tool on LinkedIn. Write a short paragraph on why you are reaching out. Here is an example:

> Hello Sir/Madam,
>
> I am looking to expand my connection in the field of pharmaceutical ethics and compliance. I saw that you work for XYZ organization. I would love to connect, hear about your experiences, and gain advice on how to leverage my medical degree for this career. Can we do a virtual coffee?
>
> Sincerely,
> Your name

Set up a Zoom virtual coffee. Your goal is to give your time to get their time. Hear their story. Then share your story and what you are looking for. Genuinely get to know the person. Keep in touch with them every month. You will create a lasting impression and be first on their call list when there are future openings within their organization.

About Dr. SK

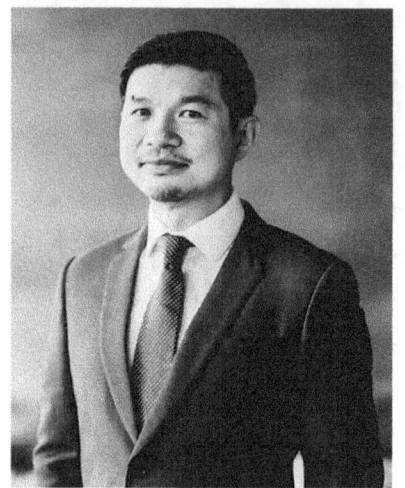

Swee Kheng Khor, MD, MRCP, MPH, MPP earned his Doctor of Medicine degree from the National University of Malaysia (UKM) in 2006, and subsequently obtained a Membership of the Royal College of Physicians of the UK in 2011. He earned a Master of Public Health degree from the University of California, Berkeley in 2016, and a Master of Public Policy degree from the University of Oxford in 2020. He has 15 years of progressively senior roles in the public, pharmaceutical, academic, and non-profit sectors on three continents.

Dr. SK was a doctor for the Ministry of Health, Malaysia from 2006-2010. He was Medical Manager for Abbott Laboratories, Singapore from 2010-2012. He worked with AbbVie Pharmaceuticals as Associate Director for the Middle East and North Africa, Director for China, Director for the Middle East and Africa, and Ethics and Compliance Director for EEMEA from 2013-2019. Currently, Dr. SK is a consultant for several international organizations. He is also a columnist for several media outlets and think tanks across five countries.

Chapter 17

Planetary Doctor

Overview

Job Title	Planetary Doctor / Planetary Healer / Planetary Health Advocate
Salary Range	This is a new field. No salary ranges were found
Education and Training/ Skills/ Training	Verbal and written communication skills, leadership skills, program and project management skills
Projected Job Growth	See the Future Growth section for trends in the industry

Disclaimer: The views and opinions expressed in this chapter do not necessarily reflect the views of the author.

What is a Planetary Doctor?

Planetary health is the integrated vision of health for the people and the planet. In 2015, the Rockefeller Foundation and The Lancet launched the concept of planetary health as a new discipline in global health, referring to it as the completed well-being of the human race and all ecosystems on which it depends.[128] Globally, there is decreased access to clean water, diminished air quality, more frequent natural disasters, and threatened food production.[129] The consequences of environmental degradation fuel the spread of infectious diseases such as Ebola, Zika, and severe acute respiratory syndrome (SARS). It also progresses malnutrition, heat-related illnesses, and vector-borne diseases.[130]

Planetary doctors are the stewards and frontline solution to planetary health. They have a distinctive capability to appreciate health challenges and communicate planetary strategies that individuals can take to safeguard their health and the health of their environment.[131,132]

The Clinicians for Planetary Health (C4PH) was recently formed by a select group of global clinicians who advocate for planetary health through lifestyle modifications. They educate patients on behavior and lifestyle modifications that can improve individual health as well as improving under-resourced populations and future generations by protecting world ecosystems.[129]

Sample Case

Dr. Renzo Guinto earned his Doctor of Medicine degree from the University of the Philippines. Dr. Renzo shared his story:

> I was a reluctant medical student. I never even imagined that I would be a medical doctor. It was even a joke in my home that Renzo was quite afraid of blood. I ended up going to medical school because there was this program in the University of the Philippines where, if you were in the top 40 of the nearly 70,000 high school students from across the Philippines and took the University of the Philippines' College Admission Test (UPCAT), then you got invited into a fast-track program by the College of Medicine. So, I got a letter asking if I was interested in the seven-year medical program. I thought, maybe this is God telling me I should be pursuing a career in health.
>
> I still vividly remember when I encountered the field of public health and global health. I realized I could still be a doctor, just not a doctor for individual patients. I could become a doctor for society, for the community, for a bigger population, and for public health. It was quite attractive to me because it is the confluence of clinical medicine and other disciplines such as the social sciences. I love politics and understanding culture. I love the humanities and the creativity of art. In public health, the patient is not the individual, but society at large. I can unleash my myriad interests. It is not just clinical work,

but also seeing through a political lens and understanding economics, culture, and human behavior.

Physicians have been highly regarded in society because of their medical training and oath. Healing will forever be embedded in our DNA. Whether you end up in business or the humanities, the healing mission will always be there. We need to be constantly reminded of our responsibility, privilege, and mission that is bestowed upon us.[131]

Dr. Renzo earned his Doctor of Public Health degree from Harvard University. He was named an Emerging Voice in Global Health by Health Systems Global. He stated:

One of the advocacies I espouse is climate change and environmental health. I saw Al Gore's documentary, *An Inconvenient Truth.* I was bothered by ice melting and polar bears getting dehydrated. But more importantly, I was bothered by people getting sick because of a warming planet. This is the global health problem of the 21st century — a continuously warming planet, sea level rising, and mosquitoes spreading around the world. The changing environmental conditions will have grave impacts on the health of human populations, especially the poor and the underprivileged. We need to address these issues. I cannot be a doctor for humans alone. I need to be a doctor for the planet as well.[131]

Roles and Responsibilities

Globally, over 700 clinicians have formally signed the C4PH Initiative. Over 30 medical associations and healthcare organizations have co-signed and partnered with The Lancet in committing to acting on planetary health.[129,132] Dr. Renzo shared his perspective:

We cannot detach ourselves from the health of Mother Earth. The field of public health improves the health of the world. We have added 30 years of life expectancy for the past 100 years, unfortunately, at the expense of the planet. We have a climate crisis. We have humanized our natural environments. Cities keep growing and emitting all these noxious pollutants to the atmosphere. Meanwhile, the food system that is nourishing us is also making us fat and sick. Two billion people on earth are over-consuming; they are overweight and obese. One billion people on earth are under-consuming;

they are malnourished. The same food system is emitting carbon and utilizing water, soil, and energy. The COVID-19 pandemic, in my opinion, started from an interaction of a human being and an animal. This is the time for us to reassess even our relationships with animals. These are just some of the planetary health challenges.[131]

Planetary doctors have four broad responsibilities. First, they do research to understand and analyze the complex nature of planetary health problems. Planetary health commits to evidence-based solutions. Since planetary health problems – climate change and biodiversity loss – require a transdisciplinary approach, planetary doctors collaborate with scientists and practitioners from various disciplines and sectors.

Second, they serve as communicators who share the message of planetary health to the community. Because planetary health is a new concept, they frequently speak at conferences, workshops, podcasts, and webinars. They engage, educate, and convince their audiences about the importance of taking care of the environment as part of the public solution. They write for journals, websites, and blogs. They develop outreach materials to create awareness about health and environmental benefits of planetary health actions and share stories of success.[130,132]

Third, they mobilize communities to rally around positive change for planetary health. They lead grassroots events and initiatives to promote community actions such as advocating for bike lanes, organizing farmer's markets, and adopting clean renewable energy.[2] Planetary health emphasizes working closely with indigenous communities, which for millennia have recognized the inextricable link between our health and the health of the planet. Dr. Renzo stated:

> We must connect with our roots, with indigenous communities who remind us that Mother Earth is not something we own and consume, but something we are merely a part of.[131]

Finally, planetary doctors conduct advocacy to influence policy and systems. Ultimately, planetary health problems can only be solved by changing policies and transforming systems – whether they pertain to food, water, energy, cities, forests, or other aspects of the ecosystem. Therefore, planetary doctors must constantly work with policy makers, politicians, and business leaders to translate planetary health knowledge into sustainable changes that can improve the health of the current generation and those that are yet to come.

Planetary doctors also build communities. Dr. Renzo reiterated:

I am very much involved in building planetary health communities in the Philippines. It is called pH2. We are building a community in Southeast Asia because, at the end of the day, the Philippines is not working in isolation anymore. We are part of a global inter-regional community. Several scholars and professionals from across the region are working together to build a robust and vibrant community for advancing the field of planetary health in the region.[131]

Skills, Education, Certification, and Training

There is no formal education, certification, or training needed to transition into this field. Two of the most critical skill sets to master for this career are verbal and written communication skills. Dr. Renzo explained:

In planetary health, you must possess the ability to tell stories to convey complex ideas in simple ways. It is also important to have the ability to convert ideas into practical solutions that can be disseminated, digested, and adopted by different audiences.[131]

Another skill to acquire and develop is leadership skills. Dr. Renzo stated:

Planetary doctors must be able to bring people together, articulate a vision, and inspire communities to act.[131]

Finally, because planetary health problems require transdisciplinary and cross-sectoral solutions, planetary doctors must develop skills for collaborative research, with the ability to connect the dots over a wide range of issues.[131]

Pros and Cons

Some advantages to becoming a planetary doctor are:

1. Global partnerships. You work with the world's top planetary health experts from renowned institutions and organizations. Your partnerships will propel you to reach greater heights and will open doors for speaking engagements, projects, and programs.

2. Teamwork. As much as your career hinges on your independent drive and motivation to find opportunities, most of your assignments occur with other highly esteemed professionals. Working well in groups is of utmost importance in tackling challenging global issues.

3. New field. Planetary health is in its infancy. The opportunities are limitless. This field is a blank canvas. You can utilize your creativity and innovativeness to make this career work for you.

4. Saving the planet. Your impact is powerful. Your ideas and actions will potentially save the Earth, including plants, animals, and human lives. Future generations will appreciate your efforts.

Some challenges to becoming a planetary doctor are:

1. Compensation is challenging. If you want to work full-time, you will need to start your own business as a planetary doctor. This includes marketing, publicity, content writing, financials, and budgeting. Multiple revenue streams may be required to make this career sustainable. Fortunately, you can work with other established planetary doctors to mentor you along the way.

2. Connections count. Your work will depend on your global connections and credibility. Your relationships provide opportunities for your first project and program. Your professional connections will help spread the news about your new venture.

Future Growth

Planetary health is a hot topic. Life expectancy has increased more than 20 years over the past 50 years. The total number of individuals living in extreme poverty has dropped by 700 million in the past 30 years.[133] Humans are living longer and better lives. Human health is affecting planetary health and vice versa. The need for subject-matter experts in this field is evident. The demand for educated, well-intentioned, and determined individuals is increasing, yet the supply is low.

Now What?

1. Find your niche in planetary health. You can focus on climate change and its health impacts or find solutions to transform the global diet to become both nutritious and low carbon. Or you can help design cities that are health-promoting and environmentally sustainable. There are nine planetary boundaries: climate crisis, ocean acidification, ozone depletion, nitrogen-phosphorus cycle, freshwater use, deforestation/land changes, biodiversity loss, particle overload of the atmosphere, and chemical pollution.[134]

2. Read and learn about your niche. Read journals, articles, magazines, and books. Listen to podcasts, webinars, and conferences. Take additional coursework or attain an advanced degree to increase your credibility in the public eye. Be a subject-matter expert in your chosen niche.

3. Find a planetary doctor mentor. Dr. Renzo has extended an invitation to mentor individuals who are new to the field of planetary health. Connect with me on social media and I will bridge an introduction. He stated:

   > Part of my work is to mentor the next generation of planetary healers. Learning does not happen only in the classroom; it also comes from relationships.[131]

4. Create content. Be creative and innovative, but factual and data-driven with your content. Submit your content to educational magazines and journals. You are laying the groundwork for your digital footprint and establishing your name in the planetary health field. This, in turn, will open up possibilities and opportunities.

About Dr. Renzo

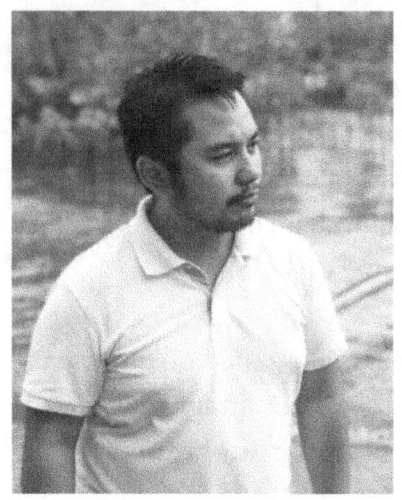

Renzo Guinto, MD, DrPH is one of the most exciting and innovative voices for the new discipline of planetary health. Dr. Renzo is Chief Planetary Doctor of pH Lab – a think tank for advancing the health of both people and the planet. He is Associate Professor of the Practice of Global Public Health and Inaugural Director of the Global Health Program of the St. Luke's Medical Center College of Medicine – William H. Quasha Memorial in the Philippines.

Dr. Renzo is an Obama Foundation Asia-Pacific Leader, Aspen Institute New Voices Fellow, and Climate Reality Leader under the initiative of former US Vice President Al Gore. He is a member of several high-level international groups including: Lancet–Chatham House Commission on Improving Population Health post COVID-19 (University of Cambridge); Lancet One Health Commission (University of Oslo); Advisory Council of Global Health 50/50 (University College London); Advisory Board of Climate Cares (Imperial College London); Editorial Advisory Board of The Lancet Planetary Health; and Forum on Climate Change and Health of the World Innovation Summit for Health (Qatar Foundation). He has served as a consultant for various organizations including World Health Organization, World Bank, USAID, International Organization for Migration, Health Care Without Harm, Philippine Department of Health, Chilean Ministry of Health, and Institute of Tropical Medicine in Belgium.

Dr. Renzo earned his Doctor of Public Health degree from Harvard University and his Doctor of Medicine degree from the University of the Philippines, Manila. He received further training from the University of Oxford, University of Copenhagen, University of the Western Cape in South Africa, and East-West Center in Hawaii. In 2020, he was included by Tatler Magazine in its Gen. T List of 400 leaders of tomorrow who are shaping Asia's future. He was named as Emerging Voice in Global Health by Health Systems Global, Emerging Leader by the World Heart Federation, and Raffles Fellow by the National University of Singapore. Dr. Renzo has lectured in nearly 50 countries; published more than 100 articles in scientific journals, books, and popular media; and directed and produced short films that communicate the message of planetary healing to the world.

Chapter 18

Professor

Overview

Job Title	Professor
Salary Range	Average annual income in the US: $100,021. Ranges from $51,000 (10th percentile) to $200,000 (90th percentile)[135]
Education/Training	At least a master's degree for community college and a doctorate degree for 4-year college and university. On-the-job training available. Entry-level starts as a visiting professor, progresses to an associate professor, and culminates as a full-time professor
Skills/Talents	Verbal and communication skills, mentoring skills, public speaking skills
Sample companies	Any public or private college or university
Projected Job Growth	Approximately 9% increase projected in the US from 2019-2029[136]

What is a Professor?

A Professor is someone who is an expert in some art or science. He/she is a teacher of the highest rank.[137] Professors work at colleges and post-secondary educational institutions. In northern Europe, the title of professor is the highest academic rank at the university. The title varies with experience from associate, full-time, and emeritus professor in the US and Canada.[137,138]

Sample Case

Dr. Kenneth Hartigan-Go earned his Doctor of Medicine degree from the University of the Philippines and completed his Internal Medicine specialty at the Philippine General Hospital (PGH), Philippines. He started teaching as Clinical Associate Professor of the Department of Internal Medicine at PGH in 1991-1992. He was subsequently named Assistant Professor and then promoted to Professor III for the Department of Pharmacology and Toxicology at the University of the Philippines College of Medicine from 1990-2005. Dr. Kenneth stated:

> I was invited to join the faculty of medicine to teach under that department. I spent 15 years in the College of Medicine teaching, doing clinical practice, and internal medicine.[139]

Dr. Kenneth was the former Head of the Stephen Zuellig Graduate School of Development Management at the Asian Institute of Management. His training ground was his practice of internal medicine and public health services. He shared:

> Being a clinician was not enough for me. I headed the Adverse Drug Reaction Monitoring Program for the Philippine Government in partnership with the Australian Assistance for International Development. Later, I was invited to join the Bureau of Food and Drugs in the Philippine Department of Health as Deputy Director working in the National Drug Policy Program. I was then invited to join the Asian Institute of Management, promoting development management. The way I want to create change in the world is by motivating and inspiring students.[139]

Roles and Responsibilities

A professor's responsibilities fall under three categories: planning, implementation, and evaluation. Primarily, professors plan lessons while staying informed on developments and innovations within their fields. They develop a curriculum for their course while ensuring university standards and policies. Dr. Kenneth stated:

> I was tasked with developing and designing courses, both executive short courses and master's degree courses. Our school is focused on development. We have two programs. One is called Master of Development Management degree. It is a 32-year-old program that deals with social entrepreneurs,

development investors, and governmental officers. We work with non-governmental organizations (NGOs). We measure the social return of investment and the impact on the community as it aligns with its sustainable development goal.

On the other hand, there is another master's program where I am the academic program director for the pioneering course called Masters in Disaster Risk and Crisis Management. We are developing a cadre of leaders in the government, private business sector, and NGOs to work on the disaster management cycle from preparation to prevention to response to recovery and rehabilitation. Students have to understand how business and society work together to create the narrative and conversation with the right people and create change. They must learn the language of disaster, the science of disaster, and how to apply ethics in making decisions.[139]

Secondly, professors implement their knowledge as subject-matter experts. They teach courses and work with students to improve their knowledge and skills. They conduct and publish research to accelerate and facilitate learning. They also serve on committees in academia and in government to make recommendations based on their expertise. Dr. Kenneth practices what he teaches. From 1999-2001, he was Deputy Director of the Bureau of Food and Drugs and Manager of the National Drug Policy Program in the Philippine Department of Health. Together with the Secretary of Health, they crafted a health sector reform agenda and created FOURmula One for Health which became the guiding framework for health sector reforms.

Thirdly, professors assess and evaluate their students through grading exams, papers, and other projects. They supervise and mentor students through education to their career continuum. Other roles, such as grant writing and research achievements, depend on the educational institution and country.

Skills, Education, Certification, and Training

A master's degree is required for teaching in community colleges and a doctorate degree is required for teaching in 4-year universities. This may vary depending on the location and institution. However, subject-matter expertise is necessary to become an exemplary professor.

Being able to communicate ideas effectively through public speaking is essential. A professor's work involves speaking in front of student groups that can range from three students to hundreds of students depending on the size of the lecture halls or the course context. It is vital to develop reasonable control over tone, pitch, and pace of speech.

Furthermore, possessing a mentor mindset can set you apart from other professors. Genuine care and concern contribute to student success in life and career. A professor who actively listens and gives constructive advice can awaken a passion in a young student. Be that professor who exudes care.

Pros and Cons

Some advantages to becoming a professor are:

1. You shape future leaders. Dr. Kenneth stated:

    > Within the Asian Institute of Management, we want to produce socially responsible leaders and managers. At some point in their life and career, they must think about what contribution they want to make to society.[139]

2. You can teach the way you learned in medical school. Dr. Kenneth explained:

    > The method of teaching can be borrowed from the medical field. There, a student learns a case file with their attending doctor, sees a patient, looks at the patient's organ systems and their problems, and then summarizes a treatment plan with a holistic mindset. It is the same thing in a classroom. There is a case. We analyze it from a similar perspective. Who are the players and the stakeholders? What are the rules and what are the problems? How do they plan on addressing these problems?[139]

3. Teamwork. Dr. Kenneth emphasized the importance of teamwork. He stated:

    > The ability to get people to leave their egos behind, be willing to walk the extra mile, and create a team is crucial in learning. I think now we have to look at how to build good teamwork for functionality. [139]

4. Work/life balance. Most professors work regular office hours from 8 a.m. to 5 p.m. However, there are usually extended hours at the end of the semester for grading papers, exams,

and projects. If you choose not to work during summers, it would be a great time to spend with family.

5. Some classes are online. Online learning accelerated during COVID-19. Though it is not the medium of choice for many professors, it is essential to acquaint yourself with the online learning workflow should you be tasked with teaching online courses.

Some challenges to becoming a professor are:

1. Academic tenure takes time. Academic tenure (which exists in some countries only) is an indefinite educational appointment post that can only be terminated due to extraordinary circumstances.[140] Professors generally wait seven years to move into tenure-track positions. Tenure is mainly granted after a thorough review of the candidate's body of research, contribution to the institution, and teaching achievements.[141]

2. Entry into this career can be a challenge. Most academic positions are friendlier to those who have previous classroom experience such as teaching assistant or visiting lecturer. Most universities also look for subject-matter experts in their field of teaching.

Future Growth

According to the US Bureau of Labor Statistics, the overall employment for post-graduate or post-secondary professors is projected to grow by approximately 9% in the US from 2019 to 2029.[136] Although the projected employment growth varies by academic field, location, and years of experience, it is still greater than the average for all occupations.

It is vital to dig deep into trends of higher education. One marker is the state of the economy. For most community colleges, enrollment tends to increase during economic uncertainties. For instance, during the US recession of 2007 to 2009, there was a 33% increase in two-year college enrollment between 2006 and 2011. On the other hand, in 2010 and 2019, when the economy was healthy, many community colleges, and some universities, saw a decline in enrollment by 25%.[142]

Another trend to look out for is online education, which will continue to thrive. Currently, one-third of higher education students take at least one class online.[142] This has increased during the COVID-19 pandemic as we have seen more courses offered through online learning platforms. The new generation is accustomed to technology, and are therefore comfortable using technology to learn new knowledge and skills.

Last, but of no less importance, there is an increasing trend for competency-based education (CBE) in higher education. CBE is an educational model whereby students learn and gain skills at their own pace. This has received significant traction among students with work experience because they graduate faster and pay less money.[143]

Now What?

1. Build your teaching portfolio. Compile your teaching experiences, whether they were for workshops, seminars, or courses. Keep in mind the topics you gravitated toward.

2. Find your niche. Now is an excellent time to determine the topics you are passionate about and in which have a solid background. If you were given a chance to teach and discuss three topics to an audience, what would those topics be?

3. Look for opportunities to be a visiting lecturer. One way to maneuver yourself into the teaching world is by becoming a visiting lecturer at a university. Ask a friend or colleague who teaches at a university how to go about this process. Utilize your network and connections. Don't be afraid to ask for opportunities.

About Dr. Kenneth

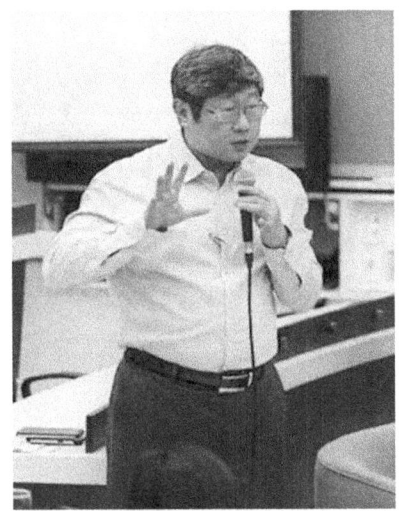

Kenneth Hartigan-Go, MD, FPCP, FACP, FRCP (Edin), FICD is an adjunct faculty member and former Head of the Stephen Zuellig Graduate School of Development Management at the Asian Institute of Management (2016-2020). He was Philippine Department of Health Undersecretary (2015-2016), Director General of Food and Drugs Administration (2012-2014), Founding Executive Director of the Zuellig Foundation (2001-2009), and Deputy Director the Bureau of Food and Drugs (1999-2001). He was a faculty member of the University of the Philippines College of Medicine (1990-2006), Ateneo School of Medicine and Public Health (2007-2010), and Asian Institute of Management (2010-2015).

He holds Doctor of Medicine degrees from the University of the Philippines College of Medicine (Philippines, 1985) and Newcastle University (United Kingdom, 1998). He is a Fellow of the Royal College of Physicians (Edinburgh), a Fellow of the American College of Physicians, Honorary Fellow of the Academy of Medicine (Singapore), Honorary Fellow of the Singapore College of Physicians (2017), and President of the Philippine College of Physicians (2017-2018).

From 2013-2016, Dr. Kenneth served as an advisor to the Chair of the Asian-Pacific Economic Cooperation's (APEC) Life Science Innovation Forum (LSIF) Executive Board. He served as a member of the WHO Global Advisory Committee on Vaccine Safety and the WHO Advisory Committee on the Safety of Medicinal Products. He is a member of the Steering Committee of the National University of Singapore Initiative for Health in Asia (NIHA) and an Expert Panel member of the Center for Regulatory Excellence based in Singapore. In the mid-2000's he was President of the Corporate Network for Disaster Response (CNDR) and a founding member of Laban Konsyumer Inc, an NGO consumer advocacy organization since 2016. He sits on the boards of Cullion Foundation Inc, Equicom Savings Bank, Maxicare Health Corporation, Generika, OML Center for Climate Change Adaptation, CARD MRI BotiCARD Inc, and is a member of the National Council of Biosafety in the Philippines. He is currently President of the International Society of Pharmacoeconomics and Outcome Research, Philippine Chapter.

Dr. Kenneth was the recipient of numerous awards including UP Alumni Association Distinguished Alumni Award for Government Service (2015); Outstanding Graduate Award, ROTC, Armed Forces of the Philippines (2012); Distinguished Fellow Award, Philippines College of Physicians (2008); Dr. Jose P. Rizal Award for Excellence as Outstanding Chinese Filipino in the Field of Medicine, the Manila Times (2008); and The Drug Information Association Outstanding Service Award, USA (2001).

Chapter 19

Quality Coordinator

Overview

Job Title	Quality Coordinator / Quality Assurance Coordinator / Quality Management Coordinator / Quality Consultant / Quality Specialist
Salary Range	Average annual income in US: $64,842. Ranges from $43,000 (10th percentile) to $96,000 (90th percentile)[144]
Education	Bachelor's degree
Training	On-the-job training available in some companies
Skills/Talents	Quality improvement, performance improvement, process improvement, attention to detail, customer service skills
Sample Companies	AbbVie, Agenus, Baxter, Bluebird Bio, Blueprint Medicines, Eli Lilly, Eurofins, Hoffmann-La Roche, Incyte Corporation, Intercept Pharmaceuticals Inc, IPSEN, Kala Pharmaceuticals, Sage Therapeutics, Seattle Genetics, Servier Pharmaceuticals, Syneos Health, ViiV Healthcare,
Projected Job Growth	Approximately 18% decline is expected in the US from 2018-2028[145]

What is a Quality Coordinator?

A quality coordinator juggles data collection and analytics to improve the organization's quality, performance, and processes. They work to implement and maintain state and federal regulatory standards and requirements in their respective industries. They work in the healthcare arenas of medical devices, pharmaceuticals, and other health service organizations. In simpler terms, a quality coordinator serves as an internal audit department.

Sample Case

Dr. Ghattas El Bassit earned his Doctor of Medicine degree from the University of Balamand, Lebanon in 2014. He immigrated to the US to be with family and pivoted to an alternative career as a quality coordinator. During the interview, Dr. Gus was raw and honest about his challenges and stated:

> I had a difficult journey. I came here looking for a fresh start. I expected things to be easier. In my mind, who would not want somebody with a medical degree or at least an equivalent of a PhD to work in the health sector? Surprisingly, nobody did. This was a huge challenge. When I had interviews, they were focused on why I left medicine. Many told me they would love to hire me, but they could not pay me what they thought I should be paid. I had to apply for a hundred jobs (not exaggerating) to get one or two interviews. But, at the end of the day, I only needed one job to make it. What was challenging and heartbreaking was, at a certain point I began thinking, did I make the wrong choice? Is there something wrong with my resume? Do I not have the proper skills to perform certain functions? For two years, I was able to do post-doctorate work in research in the Molecular Medicine Department at the University of South Florida. I went through many jobs, none of which were either compatible or paid enough for the competencies I possessed. So, for the next year and a half I went in and out of jobs, working for insurance companies, medical record review businesses, and teaching at colleges. Nothing seemed to fit until now. I work with Lion's Eye Institute for Transplant and Research as Quality Assurance Specialist in the Quality Department.[146]

Roles and Responsibilities

The quality coordinator's responsibilities fall under four categories: auditing and compliance, document management, complaints, and interdepartmental training and communication.

Quality coordinators develop and implement internal auditing practices to ensure compliance with industry standards and statutory regulations. These professionals write and shape organizational procedures and policies. They serve as resources who support auditing teams to undertake regular audits and compliance assessments. They develop quality improvement plans to monitor and continuously improve organizational compliance, resolving any issues promptly.[147,148]

Record management policies and procedures are developed and implemented by quality coordinators. They are responsible for retention and disposal of records and strict adherence to company policy on document management. They educate staff on good practices including document creation, approval, publishing, review, archive, and storage. Maintenance and continuous improvement of record management procedures is required.[148]

Quality coordinators receive incoming complaints and allocate them to the appropriate department for investigation and resolution. They develop tools and resources to standardize the investigation of complaints. By monitoring complaints, they identify areas of improvement within the organization.[148]

Interdepartmental training and communication is another important role of quality coordinators. These professionals maintain relationships with stakeholders, clients, customers, and staff. They provide support for projects from inception to completion. They facilitate meetings, workshops, and focus groups to communicate, disseminate information, and train staff to reach quality goals.[147,148]

Dr. Gus stated:

> We audit all processes from recovering corneas and tissues for transplantation to distribution to recipient patients. I will give you an example. A month ago, we traveled to the recovery sites (hospital, medical examiner's exam room, or morgue) where technicians were recovering corneas from the donors. On these trips, we audit the process of removing the corneas while preserving sterility. We also audit the shipping of the cornea. Is it labeled correctly? Is it placed in the container correctly? Is everything following standard operating procedures? We even do environmental control and monitoring to make sure we are working in a sterile environment. We audit, for instance, the phone calls to the donor's family or next of kin. Are they asking the right medical questions? Are they documenting

properly? We also audit patient medical charts to determine whether the donor is eligible to donate the gift that they are giving.[146]

Skills, Education, Certification, and Training

There is no formal education or certification required to work in quality assurance. However, a good quality coordinator requires extensive knowledge of their industry's governing institutions and agencies. Dr. Gus stated:

> You must possess a vast amount of knowledge about the governing organizations of your industry. For me, it is the Eye Bank Association of America (EBAA) and Food and Drug Administration (FDA). One of the major skills needed is people skills. You interact with a lot of people and are seen as the policemen of the organization. Whenever my team shows up at a department, the first reaction is something along the lines of, 'What did I do now?' It is important to have proper people skills to diplomatically and empathetically explain the reason for the visit. We want to avoid confrontation. There is also constant learning. Standard operating procedures change; regulations change. When COVID-19 hit, new regulations came from all agencies.[146]

Pros and Cons

Some of the advantages to becoming a quality coordinator are:

1. Some organizations train newcomers. If you are keen on learning more about quality assurance, search for organizations that provide on-the-job training. Showing that you are an avid learner and expressing strong interest to the management team will put you in a better position in gaining employment.

2. There is potential for internal growth within your organization. You can start as a quality coordinator and move up through the organization, being promoted to quality supervisor, quality manager, and quality director. Dr. Gus recalled:

> The toughest part is getting your foot in the door. Once you are in, most of the time you are going to impress. And when you impress, you are always up for promotions.[146]

3. The skills you develop in a quality assurance position are transferrable. Quality control is universal. Once you have quality assurance experience, you can shift from one healthcare organization to another without extensive entry barriers. You can redirect your skills and knowledge within a specific industry to a wide variety of healthcare organizations and locations.

4. Your organization's product or service can change lives. Dr. Gus stated:

> We had a young lady come in who had a genetic disorder where her cornea was clouded. She could not see anything. She successfully received one of the corneas we recovered. She is now the spokesperson for the company. She can now see even small details because of her transplant surgery. It is beautiful to witness the gift of sight.[146]

Some challenges to becoming a quality coordinator are:

1. If you have no experience, you start from square one. You will need to start as a quality coordinator before moving on to the ranks of quality supervisor, quality manager, and quality director.

2. You will be the expert on company policies and procedures. As the quality coordinator and later the quality manager, you must understand and embody your company's policies and procedures in their entirety. Dr. Gus said:

> At least four to five times a day, someone comes up to me and asks, 'Hey, are we supposed to be doing this?' Or, 'Is it okay to do that?' You will gain knowledge and build on it within this job.[146]

Future Growth

Unfortunately, there is an estimated downward trend of approximately 18% in the US from 2018 to 2028 for quality assurance professionals.[145] This trend may be due to a shift to digital health, machine learning, and automation. The rise of transformational technology will cause systems to automatically note mistakes and alter algorithms to improve outcomes. This change will decrease the frequency of audits, which will lead to less demand for human capital to conduct audits.

Now What?

1. Find a connection. LinkedIn is your best friend. Network. Search for a "Quality Coordinator," "Quality Manager," "Quality Director" in your area, and "Connect." When sending that invitation for a connection, always "Add a Note." Express your interest in why you are reaching out to this individual. Be keen to learn about their story. Share your story and aspirations. Your message should look something like this:

   > Hello Sir/Madam,
   >
   > I am looking to transition to the field of quality assurance. I see that you work for XYZ organization. I would love to hear about your experiences and receive advice on how to leverage my medical degree for this career. Can we do a virtual coffee?
   >
   > Sincerely,
   > Your name

   Set up a Zoom virtual coffee. Your goal is to give your time to get their time. Hear their story. Then, share your story and what you are looking for. Genuinely get to know the person. Keep in touch with them every month. You will create a lasting impression and be first on their call list when there are future openings within their organization.

2. Apply. This career is about putting your best foot forward and applying to several organizations. Some organizations will offer training, but it may be difficult to determine these organizations in the beginning. So, the recipe for entering this career is apply, apply, apply. When asked to share his last piece of advice, Dr. Gus stated:

   > You need to understand that, as a non-physician, you are going to get a lot of rejections. You must be humble enough to say, 'Okay, I am going to accept that, but I will keep on going.' So, do not stop. Perseverance is key. It might seem challenging at first, and a lot of times, the future may seem dark. You may have to apply to a hundred places, just as if you are applying for residency to get matched. It only takes one yes to change your entire future and career path.[146]

About Dr. Gus

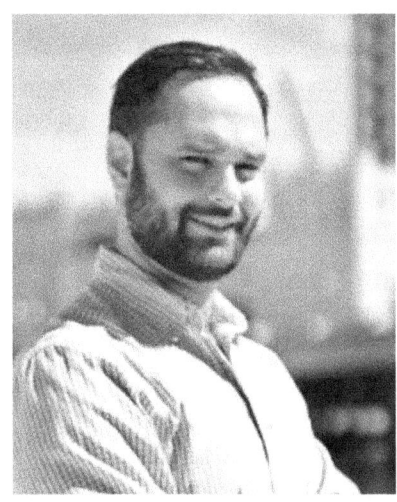

Dr. Ghattas El Bassit earned a Doctor of Medicine degree from the University of Balamand, Lebanon in 2014. He worked as a primary care physician at Proud Lebanon, a non-profit organization in Beirut, in 2015. He worked as Postdoctoral Fellow and Research Assistant for the Molecular Medicine Department at the University of South Florida in Tampa, Florida from 2015-2017. He became Quality Assurance Specialist for MSLA – a United Healthcare Group Affiliate – in Florida from 2017-2018, and Adjunct Professor at Hillsborough Community College and Galen College for Nursing in 2018. Since 2019, he has been Quality Assurance Specialist at Lion's Eye Institute for Research and Transplant.

In his free time, he is a yoga and meditation instructor. He is also learning about aromatherapy, herbology, and alternative medicine.

Chapter 20

Ship Physician

Overview

Job Title	Cruise Ship Physician
Salary Range	Average annual income in the US: $96,000 (without commission). Ranges from $90,000 to $132,000[149]
Education	MD (International Medical Graduate-friendly)
Training	ACLS, BLS, PALS, ATLS. See Skills, Education, Certification and Training section
Skills/Talents	Verbal and written communication skills, clinical skills, management skills, risk assessment skills
Sample companies	Azamara, Carnival Cruise Line, Celebrity Cruises, Crystal Cruises, Cunard, Disney Cruise Line, Norwegian Cruise Line, Oceania Cruises, Regent Seven Seas Cruises, Royal Caribbean International, Seabourn, Silversea Cruises, Viking Cruises
Projected Job Growth	See the Future Growth section for trends in the industry

What is a Cruise Ship Physician?

A cruise ship physician is a physician who practices medicine aboard a cruise ship. These physicians are responsible for the basic and emergency medical management of the crew and passengers on board the ship.

Sample Case

Dr. Alex R. Guevara, my late father, was the first Filipino cruise ship physician for Royal Caribbean International and Celebrity Cruises.[150] Doc Alex, as people called him, earned his Doctor of Medicine degree from West Visayas State University College of Medicine, Philippines in 1979 and completed his formal surgery training at Iloilo Doctors' Hospital, Iloilo City, Philippines in 1984.

My family immigrated to the United States in September 1998. Doc Alex worked as a surgical technician for a tertiary hospital in McAllen, Texas. Ultimately, a good friend referred him to Premier Cruise Line where he began working as a ship physician. As cruise ships bear an international flag and sail in international waters, he was able to use his Philippine physician's license. Cruise ships were not strict with their requirements back then and he was able to use his emergency and surgery experiences to meet their clinical requirements.

Doc Alex worked in the cruise ship industry from 1999 until 2020. Our family moved to Florida in 2001 to be closer to Port of Tampa, Florida. He worked with companies such as Premier Cruise Line, Celebrity Cruise Line, Carnival Cruise Line, Royal Caribbean International, and Norwegian Cruise Line.

Roles and Responsibilities

A cruise ship physician sounds like a dream job, even a vacation, but the position actually holds an immense amount of responsibility. Cruise ship physicians are responsible for the health, well-being, and lives, on average, of 5,000 people (crew and passengers) per cruise. The toughest part of this career is the accountability for decision-making, especially for senior doctors, who have the capability of disembarking patients and referring them to land-based facilities. This involves turning the ship around, allowing an airlift, or changing the itinerary, depending on the severity of the emergency. Ship doctors need to make sound, evidence-based medical decisions that may involve life and death situations. Their decisions can save lives and yet cost the company thousands of dollars.

Generally, cruise ship physicians see approximately 10-20 patients per day depending on the cruise itinerary, sailing conditions, and age demographic of the passengers. They evaluate and treat emergency medical, surgical, gynecological, and pediatric health problems of passengers and crew members. They deal with a wide array of medical conditions from non-infectious gastroenterology issues, motion sickness, fractures, lacerations, myocardial infarction, and stroke to name a few. They perform minor procedures such as incision and drainage, wound suturing, reduction of simple dislocations, splinting and immobilization procedures, blood transfusions and, of course, take turns during emergencies in leading the Advance Cardiac Life Support procedures and emergency airway treatment.[151]

A cruise ship's medical facility must adhere to the American College of Emergency Physicians (ACEP) standards. It is often located on a lower deck. It contains one hospital bed for every 1,000 passengers and one to two intensive care unit (ICU) beds. It is equipped for simple laboratory procedures, x-ray services, and mini-pharmacy services. It also has minor surgical equipment, oxygen tanks and respirators, and EKG machines. It contains all basic equipment found in a medical ICU such as cardiac monitors, ventilators, and defibrillators.[152]

The medical department is the smallest department on the cruise ship, yet one of the most important. It is composed of two to three doctors, three to five registered nurses, and a medical secretary. The senior doctor is the head of the department and in charge of all the junior doctors and nurses. The junior doctor mainly oversees the nurses and the medical secretary. These management responsibilities may vary depending on individual cruise line policies and procedures.

Skills, Education, Certification, and Training

Cruise ship physicians must hold a diploma from an accredited school of medicine. They carry their country's physician license to work in international waters. They have at least two years of post-graduate/post-registration clinical experience in general, intensive care unit (ICU) or emergency medicine. A board certification in emergency medicine, family medicine, or internal medicine is an advantage.[152]

In addition, they must hold a current certification in Basic Life Support (BLS), Advanced Cardiac Life Support (ACLS), Advanced Trauma Life Support (ATLS), and Pediatric Advanced Life Support (PALS). They must be willing to learn basic laboratory and x-ray procedures.

Pros and Cons

Some of the advantages to becoming a cruise ship physician are:

1. Commission. Depending on the cruise line, you receive a monthly base pay and a percentage of medical revenue for each cruise. Commission is derived from in-office medical consults, after-hour consults, diagnostics, procedures, and medication sales.

2. Couples' contracts. Most cruise companies will match contracts if you sign on as a married couple. They accommodate couples by contracting them on the same ship and have their sign-on and sign-off dates as close to each other as possible. Doc Alex and Doc Mergie, my parents, were able to work together in the same ship during the same months for several years. They worked and vacationed together.

3. Short office hours. When you are on duty, you regularly have two to three office hours in the morning and two to three office hours in the afternoon. Most of your patients, either crew or passenger, will see you during your office hours. However, there are after-hour emergencies as well.

4. Malpractice insurance is often covered by the cruise company. Lawsuits generally arise from short term injuries which do not have long term consequences. Hence, the ship physician is unlikely to be the victim of a lawsuit.[152]

5. You are an officer. You get three (sometimes three and half) epaulettes (stripes) on your uniform. In context, the captain, chief engineer, hotel manager, staff captain and staff chief engineer receive four stripes.[151] Being an officer allows you access to passenger areas when you are in uniform. There are other benefits like lodging, dining, and gift shop discount privileges mentioned below.

6. Travel while you work. It is no secret that a ship physician can request that his family travel with him for an unlimited amount of time during his contract. The prices range from free (if they stay in the ship physician's cabin) to 40% off of the total cruise cost (if they have their own cabin) depending on the cruise line. This includes lodging, free food (except for specialty restaurants) and entertainment. Doc Alex frequently requested that our family join him when he was on board. Our family has visited over 30 countries over the past 20 years.

7. The ship docks at several ports depending on the ship's itinerary. You visit a different city or country each day while at port. On your days off, you are free to roam the city with permission from the staff captain. Keep in mind you must return to the ship a couple of hours before the ship sails or the ship will leave you behind.

8. Lodging is included. With officer status, you are entitled to your own private one-bed cabin with a window (sometimes a lounge area depending on the cruise line), but no balcony. An assigned room steward cleans your room and bathroom and collects and delivers your laundry daily. The ship also provides free toiletries.

9. Unlimited free food and entertainment. You have access to daily buffet food from the passenger food hall, sit down dining in the passenger dining hall, and buffet food from the crew mess or the officer dining hall. You may attend the nightly shows with the other passengers as long as you are in evening uniform.

10. You wear a uniform. You do not have to worry about what to wear daily. You are supplied with a number of day and evening uniforms. Laundry is free for officers.

11. You do not need to know how to swim. There is no swimming requirement to be able to work as a medical staff of a cruise ship.

Some challenges to becoming a cruise ship physician are:

1. You are away from family. Contracts vary from four months to six months, with two months of unpaid vacation time between contracts. This may be difficult for those with young children. Doc Alex always considered being away from family the hardest part of working in the cruise ship industry. However, he found a silver lining in every situation. On his two months off, our whole family endeavored to make memorable experiences such as vacationing together in the Philippines.

2. Accountability for decision making. When dealing with an emergency case, where the patient needs to be evacuated, the senior doctor must effectively communicate to the captain the necessity for the disembarkation and the evacuation process. Disembarking a passenger causes financial and psychological burden to the passenger and the ship. It can even change the ship's itinerary.

3. You will be on call for 24 hours every other day. You carry a telephone daily. If there are two ship physicians, you work every other day. You are free on opposite days and may visit ports of call.

4. Ship contract rotations. Unless you have seniority and several years of experience, you often do not have a say on which ship you will be contracted with. You will likely rotate on different ships with the same cruise line. A new ship means a new culture and new co-workers. You also deal with crew members of more than 60 different nationalities. You will need to be resilient and able to work within this dynamically changing setting.

5. Navigating around the ship is a feat. It is vital to understand your way around the ship, especially during emergencies. You and your team run weekly timed drills for emergencies to make sure you are abreast of required skills. You must know your way to and from your assigned muster station. Doc Alex always studied the ship map when he signed on to a new ship. He kept note of the subtle nuances in designs. For example, one Norwegian ship has red carpet for the port (right) side and blue carpet for the starboard (left) side.

6. Benefits and other non-monetary compensation are scarce for independent contractors. If you work as an independent contractor, compared to an employee of the cruise line, you will not be eligible for medical insurance or 401(k) benefits. However, you will still receive a base pay and commission and other benefits mentioned above.

Future Growth

Before the COVID-19 pandemic, cruises were considered the fastest growing sector of the global travel industry. New travel destinations – coupled with a vast array of services, products, and experiences – made cruise trips a vacation of choice for passengers around the world. In 2018, the cruise ship industry was worth approximately $150 billion, of which $34.2 billion was revenue.[153] In 2019, the cruise industry hosted approximately 29.7 million passengers globally.[154]

The COVID-19 climate created new health and safety concerns on board cruise ships and they now work closely with the Cruise Lines International Association (CLIA) to enforce health measures. They are required to meet avid screening and monitoring protocols, comprehensive sanitation protocols with regular mandatory inspections, and maintain expanded onboard medical facilities with increased medical staff.[152]

Fortunately, passengers are still excited about cruising. A recent survey by CLIA showed that 82% of cruisers still want to book a cruise for their next vacation. Another poll by Cruisecritic.com showed that 75% were interested in cruising post COVID-19 pandemic.[153] The outlook for 2021 and onward shows a united cruise ship industry ready to cater to passengers safely.

Now What?

1. Gather all necessary requirements. Find a way to meet all requirements, especially clinical experience. If you practiced another medical specialty, contact the hospital you worked with to document the number of hours you spent in the emergency field. The documentation sample may write, "I certify that Dr. Smith has completed 100 hours in the emergency room of the XYZ Hospital from January 1, 2021 to March 1, 2021." Make sure that your documentation is written on hospital letterhead and signed by the Chief Medical Officer.

2. Complete your ACLS, BLS, PALS, and ATLS certifications. Applications with completed certifications are better received than applications without them. You may have to pay out-of-pocket for the initial completion, but once you get the contract, your renewal will be paid by the company.

3. Apply on the cruise line website. Your best approach is to apply online for the position. It helps to know someone in the cruise industry, but you are still expected to go through the online application.

About Dr. Alex

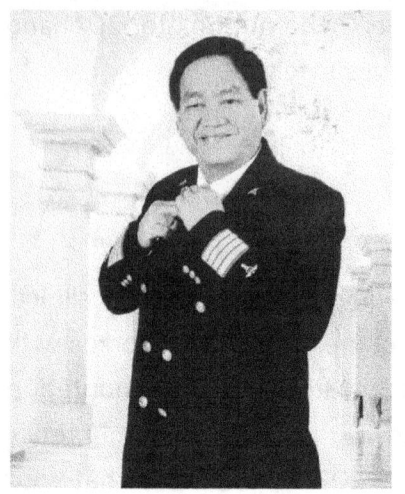

Dr. Alex R. Guevara earned his Doctor of Medicine degree from West Visayas State University College of Medicine (WVSU-COM) in Iloilo City, Philippines. He was a member of the Pioneer Class of 1979 and a founding member of the Order of Asclepius. He completed his post-graduate internship at Philippine General Hospital in Manila, Philippines in 1980 and his General Surgery residency at Iloilo Doctors' Hospital in Iloilo City, Philippines in 1984. He worked as a surgeon alongside his wife, Dr. Mergie Socorro Guevara, an anesthesiologist, for 16 years at West Visayas State University Medical Center, Iloilo Doctors' Hospital, Iloilo Mission Hospital, and St. Paul's Hospital.

As a physician, Doc Alex was known for his generosity and giving heart. He served the underprivileged Filipino population of Iloilo City and volunteered on multiple medical missions throughout the central Philippine region. He was active with Rotary Club and Lions Club providing medical resources and tools for the people of Iloilo City.

Doc Alex was renowned for his leadership and dedication to his beloved Filipino community. A full-time Associate Professor and Department Chairman in Physiology at his alma mater, founding President of the WVSU-COM Alumni Association, and President of the WVSU-COM Faculty Association, he was committed to the growth and development of the physician profession in the Philippines. He was twice voted to membership of the University Board of Regents and became President of the Physiology Society of the Philippines.

Doc Alex and Doc Mergie immigrated to the US with their three children in 1998. Working as a cruise ship physician for over 20 years, his resolve to serve patients globally was unwavering. He was employed by several cruise lines including Premier Cruises, Celebrity Cruises, Royal Caribbean Cruise Lines, Carnival Cruise Lines, and Norwegian Cruise Lines from 1999 until the time of his death on April 30, 2020.

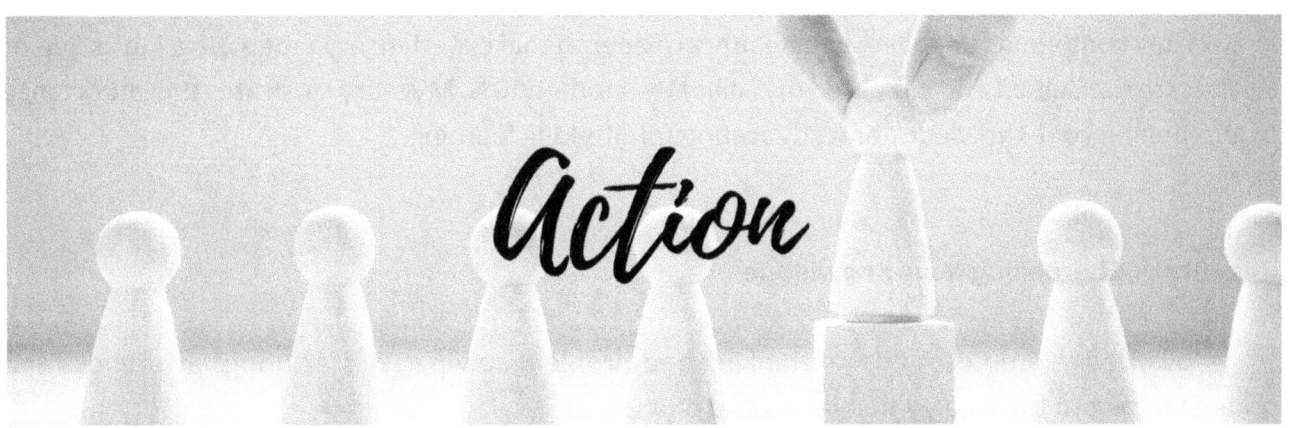

Chapter 21

Sharpen Your Knowledge

The eagle eats only fresh prey. Unlike scavengers, the eagle will starve rather than devour dead prey. [155] Always start fresh with comprehensive, well-researched information. Stay abreast of current data. Forego obsolete processes and methods. Always sharpen your knowledge.

Knowledge refers to the theoretical or practical familiarity, awareness, or understanding of a subject.[156] Learning increases intelligence. Knowledge improves mental ability. Sharpening your knowledge provides cognitive mental exercise by stimulating brain functions responsible for concentration and critical analysis.[157]

Sharpening my knowledge and upskilling were integral parts of my career development. In 2017, when I decided not to pursue a career in medicine, I made a crucial pivot to differentiate myself from my colleagues. I was working and taking classes full time. Fortunately, the university was offering online courses for a Master of Science in Health Informatics degree. After two years, I completed my master's degree and received a job offer a couple of months before graduation. My salary jumped $20,000 from attaining that additional degree. In 2020, I upskilled again by completing a Certified Professional in Healthcare Information and Management Systems (CPHIMS) certification.

In 2021, my continuous upskilling and healthcare operational experiences landed me a job as Senior Healthcare Consultant and increased my salary by another 60%. My story illustrates the importance of sharpening your knowledge and advocating for life-long learning.

Benefits of Sharpening Your Knowledge

Knowledge promotes critical thinking and problem-solving skills. It brings awareness and understanding to the what, when, and whys of a topic.

1. Know WHAT to say and how to react to other individuals. Expanding your knowledge allows you to participate in insightful conversations. It adds to the repertoire of information you draw from in responding thoughtfully to other individuals. For example, reading this book will give you knowledge about alternative careers to traditional medicine. When asked to advise other international medical graduates, you will be able to converse matter-of-factly about career path options.

2. Know WHEN to speak to other individuals. Knowledge about trends and future projections promotes critical thinking about when to act in situations. Knowledge provides foresight for strategic action, offering new angles to an old perspective. For example, knowing that there is an increasing trend in healthcare informatics and healthcare analytics allows for wise decisions on investing in this field.

3. Know the WHY and the reasoning behind your statements. Knowledge explains circumstances. It promotes the practice of reasoning and enhances your ability to solve problems. It promotes viability for high-probability, high-impact actions. For instance, knowledge about the world's aging population and the accommodations needed for an aging population explains the why of home health services.

Finding Ways to Sharpen Your Knowledge

The importance of sharpening your knowledge is vital to career development and advancement. Knowledge can be acquired through various methods, but for this chapter we will discuss learning through reading, courses/webinars, and documentaries/docuseries.[156]

1. Learning through reading. Reading books, newspapers, and articles has historically been one of the most utilized forms of learning. Now, with widespread access to technology,

information is readily available and at our fingertips. You want to read as much as you can about relevant topics that pertain to your new career. Be vigilant and consistent in fact-checking what you read online.

2. Learning through courses. Online courses are another vehicle of learning. You want to show future employers and clients that you are a subject-matter expert. Taking additional courses and earning certifications add credibility to your expertise. Here are examples of reputable websites that produce quality, comprehensive, and well-researched content:

    a. Edx.org is a nonprofit educational platform founded by Harvard and MIT in 2012. It is the learning platform of choice for international organizations like Microsoft and IBM. They offer over 20,000 courses around the world in 32 languages to over 40 million learners and is utilized by nine out of ten of the highest ranked universities. Most courses are free, but a Verified Certification will cost you $49 USD or more.[158]

    b. Coursera.org is an online learning platform that partners with over 200 top universities worldwide. They offer in excess of 4,600 courses, 490 specializations, 40 certificates, 930 projects, and 24 degrees to 76 million learners. Most 4–6-week courses are free, but you pay $39 USD or more to receive Course Certification. Most two-hour guided projects start at $9.99 USD, while 4–6-month Specialization and Professional Certificates start at $39 USD a month. Master Track Certificates start at $2,000 USD, while Online Degrees start at $9,000 USD.[159]

    c. Udemy.com is another online learning platform trusted by 80% of Fortune 100 companies for employee up-skilling. They offer more than 130,000 courses in 65 languages to 35 million learners. On a sale day, courses cost $12.99.[160]

3. Learning through conferences and webinars. Conferences and webinars from reputable healthcare organizations provide an excellent avenue for learning. They create a nurturing environment to amass expansive knowledge in a short time. It is essential to find time to digest and internalize your newfound knowledge. Take time to reread your notes after the conference or webinar. Take time to research the topics or discussions you question. Be a proactive learner.

CHALLENGE 7

Ultimately, the primary purpose of knowledge is action. Utilize the methods of learning mentioned above and apply them. Read one article and watch one webinar this week with direct relevance to your chosen field. Take action to sharpen your knowledge.

Chapter 22

Select Your Mentors

The baby eagle is trained by its mother to fly by pushing it out of the nest. The mother eagle then removes layers of soft feathers from the nest, uncovering branches and thorns below. When the baby eagle comes back, it no longer has a soft haven because its home is prickled with thorns. Shrieking, it jumps out from the nest again. This process is repeated until the baby eagle flaps its wings and flies out from its high place away from the thorns.[4] Like the baby eagle, you need someone in your life who is invested in you, someone to push you out of your comfort zone and mentor you. Challenges are painful, but without them, we do not grow and develop. Select mentors who will help you through difficult times and encourage you to soar to new heights.

Mentorship is a secret to success that is not openly talked about. It is a relationship between two people that serves as a learning opportunity to share knowledge, experience, and advice that leads to development of communication, leadership, and decision-making skills in a supportive environment.[161] Mentors are a guiding light to individuals, helping them perform better and advance faster in their careers.

Benefits of Mentorship

A mentor is a knowledgeable and experienced individual who nurtures a less knowledgeable and less experienced mentee.[162] Mentors assist individuals in deciding who they want to become, what changes are needed to attain that goal, and how to use their work experiences to bring about these changes.[163] Mentors guide and support individuals through their professional journey. Benefits of mentorship include:

1. Individualized goal setting. Mentors help accelerate career growth by defining a clear path to your goals and ambitions. They help you steer your course and keep you on the right track at the right speed.

2. Improved career outcomes. According to a meta-analysis of 43 studies by Allen et al., mentored employees were compared to non-mentored employees.[164] Their results showed that mentored employees:

    a. Received more promotions.
    b. Received higher compensations.
    c. Felt more satisfaction with their careers.
    d. Felt more commitment to their careers.
    e. Believed they would advance in their careers.

3. Foster passions and develop self-awareness. Mentors offer you a new perspective about yourself. They highlight realistic views about your strengths and weaknesses through your experiences and stories. They can propel you toward your passions.

The Ideal Mentor

Seeking a mentor is not a sign of weakness. It is the opposite. A mentor will pull out the best in you and serve as an advocate for your strengths. It is about seeking an experienced and neutral perspective in a person who has previously walked in your shoes. There are several characteristics to look for in a mentor to achieve a positive outcome.

1. Someone who seeks to help people grow. You want someone who is genuinely interested in your development and dedicated to your career advancement. These individuals believe that investing in other people creates lifelong transformative relationships which are imperative to their own growth.

2. Someone who actively listens. Mentorship is based on easy and open communication. You want someone who can tolerate your problem, possess the patience to extract the core issues from your discussion, and have the clarity to help you. They must possess the ability to communicate clearly with a less experienced individual.[165,166,167]

3. Someone who follows up. A good mentor/mentee relationship is not built overnight, but develops over multiple conversations. You want someone who follows up and follows through. Avoid people who consistently cancel meetings. Find someone eager to hear about your challenges who can objectively give you insights into finding solutions.[166,166,167]

Finding Your Mentors

Consider having three mentors who you talk with regularly. Yes, there may be countless one-time mentors who come in and out of your life. There may be those who gave you an epiphany about your career. There may be those who made an impression through their books or podcasts. This is a start, but you need someone with whom you can have an ongoing discussion about your career.

Now is the time to seek a mentor who will guide you to greatness. Here are some suggested steps you can take to find a mentor to match your needs.

1. Define your specific needs. List your SMART (specific, measurable, attainable, relevant, and time-bound) goals. Write out your goals. Some thoughts to consider include, *Who do I aspire to be? Who possesses the career of my dreams?*

2. Find someone from your second to third degree connections. Second degree connections are your friends' friends, while third degree connections are your friends' friends' friends. Try your LinkedIn network, someone from work, or an individual you met at a conference. Pay attention to those fantastic individuals who already surround you. Are there individuals in your community with whom you've had an initial interaction who left a great impression?[166,167]

3. Make a request. Do not cold email for mentorship. Asking someone through a long-winded email is too much for a potential mentor to take in. But, don't be afraid to think big and make an initial connection. Be humble and open-minded. There is no harm in asking to speak with someone and learning from their experiences. Take it slow. Trust is established over time. Learn more about each other. Remember, mentorship is a two-way relationship. Your mentor will need to evaluate you and determine if you are worth their time. See if your objectives align. Then, make the big ask for mentorship.[166,167]

CHALLENGE 8

Find someone in your secondary or tertiary network. Pick three names. Send a message or a quick text. Here is an example:

Hello,

My name is ___. We met at XYZ. Your professionalism and dedication to your work inspired me. You motivate me to be better. I would love to learn more about your experiences and wondered if we can have a 15-minute phone conversation next week on one of the following dates: A, B, C. Let me know which one works best for you. Thank you in advance.

Sincerely,
Your name

CHAPTER 23

Strengthen Your Network

The eagle is loyal to its mate. The most famous courtship ritual of eagles is known as the death spiral. Two eagles soar high in the air. They lock talons. Then, they free fall together at an enormous speed.[168] This ritual will determine if the female eagle will mate with the male eagle. Once they are partners, they remain in their relationship for life. This story exemplifies the faithfulness and loyalty in our human connections.

Strengthening your network involves creating meaningful and transformative relationships within your network. Networking is one of the best career development resources one has in attaining professional success. Networking builds upon and maintains informal relationships for the purpose of a mutually beneficial sharing of resources.[169] Networking should build meaningful professional relationships.

Benefits of Networking

Creating symbiotic relationships is a natural outcome of successful networking. It is about sharing, rather than simply taking. Regular interaction within your network is vital to strengthening your relationships. Finding opportunities to help people within your network gives you leverage for reciprocal assistance in the future. Here are some of the benefits of networking:

1. Career development. Networking is an effective method of accelerating career development. Researchers agree that professional success is directly correlated with good networking skills.[170] A global LinkedIn survey was conducted in 2017 and included 15,905 LinkedIn

members across 17 countries. The survey revealed that approximately 80% of professionals consider networking an essential component of career success.[171] Often, the most connected individuals end up being the most successful in their industries and vice versa. Most positions are filled using personal connections. Approximately 70% of the sample population reported that they were hired at a company where they had a connection.[171]

2. Access to job opportunities. Networking can establish your reputation as being knowledgeable and reliable in your industry. Through your connections, you will stay abreast of the current job market and gain insight into market trends and job leads. When a job opening presents itself, your network will remember you. This increases your chances for valuable introductions and referrals. According to the LinkedIn survey mentioned above, approximately 61% of professionals stated regular interaction with their network could provide new job opportunities.[171]

3. Attain fresh ideas. Networking provides an opportunity to exchange knowledge with your peers. It will facilitate learning new business processes and industry best practices and developments. Discussing your challenges will allow opportunities for advice, guidance, and support while promoting fresh ideas and new perspectives.[172]

Finding Your Network — Who?

Networking can be a daunting task. Let us begin our networking challenge by enumerating prospective connections. Here are some examples:

1. Business associates. This is a broad category that includes individuals with whom you have interacted in your past or present career. Specifically, they are work colleagues, managers, and supervisors. This may also include customers and clients.

2. University alumni. Most universities have local chapters. Contact your university alumni association and request contact information for your local chapter officers. Connect with these local chapter leaders through social media. Sign up for their online newsletter or join their email list.

3. Individuals from your community service organizations, churches, and gyms are good places to start. There are several community service and nonprofit organizations in every locality across the US. This includes Rotary International, Kiwanis International, Lions Club, Toastmasters International, Key Club, American Cancer Society, American Heart Association,

and National 4H Council to name a few. Join organizations that reflect your personal values and interests.

Finding Your Network – How?

1. Figure out your networking style. There are many approaches to networking and there is no one-size-fits-all method. Find an approach that works for you. For instance, would you prefer networking one-on-one over coffee? Or would you choose a networking event with several attendees mingling from one group to another? Or even better, what about a combination of both one-on-one and group networking?

2. Figure out your networking setting. Join your alma mater's local alumni chapter, a community organization, or a sports league. Try volunteering with a non-profit organization. Follow their social media platforms and stay abreast of upcoming community events. Try Google searching for networking organizations in your area. For example, some networking organizations that exist in my hometown are Network After Work, Networking 4 a Cause, and Tampa Bay Business Network. These organizations have monthly networking events for professionals across various industries. Try online networking as well. Initiate the first message to a LinkedIn connection. Ask them for a one-on-one coffee.

3. Figure out a comfortable networking approach that feels natural, but don't be afraid to stray outside of your comfort zone. Network with a strategy in mind. How will you approach your new connection? I suggest starting by simply introducing yourself and stating your intention: "Hello, I am Nicole. I would like to get to know you. Tell me about yourself." The response might be, "What would you like to know?" This opens the door to a wide array of replies. You can ask, "What industry do you work in? What do you do for a career?" Always network with a goal in mind. What is your take-home after a networking event? Examples include connecting with three people at an event and taking home an insight to share with your co-workers.

4. Follow through with your networking encounters. Request business cards and send thank you emails the day after an event. Connect on social media platforms by sending a quick message, "It was wonderful connecting with you at XYZ event. Let me know when you have time for a coffee so we can continue our conversation."

CHALLENGE 9

Network with three people this week, utilizing the methods stated above. Schedule this because what gets scheduled, gets done.

CHALLENGE 10

Follow through with your three new connections next week.

References

Introduction:

1. ECFMG. (2020, March 02). International Medical graduate (IMG) Performance in the 2020 Main Residency Match. Retrieved August 1, 2020, from https://www.ecfmg.org/resources/Match2020Infographic.pdf

2. National Resident Matching Program. (2018, July). Charting Outcomes in the Match: International Medical Graduates. Retrieved October 14, 2020, from https://www.nrmp.org/wp-content/uploads/2018/06/Charting-Outcomes-in-the-Match-2018-IMGs.pdf

3. Murdock, J. (2020, July 15). Humans have more than 6,000 thoughts per day, psychologists discover. Retrieved December 02, 2020, from https://www.newsweek.com/humans-6000-thoughts-every-day-1517963

Chapter 1: Realize Your Breakthrough and Get Ready to Break Away

4. Anderson, M. (2016, April 13). 7 Career Transition Lessons We Can Learn From An Eagle. Retrieved April 12, 2020, from https://www.kickstartcareers.co.uk/blog/2016/04/13/7-career-transition-lessons-we-can-learn-from-an-eagle

5. The Editors of Encyclopaedia Britannica. (2019, December 04). Hippocratic oath. Retrieved September 01, 2020, from https://www.britannica.com/topic/Hippocratic-oath

6. Stefan Riedel (2005) Edward Jenner and the History of Smallpox and Vaccination, Baylor University Medical Center Proceedings, 18:1, 21-25. Retrieved April 12, 2020, from https://doi.org/10.1080/08998280.2005.11928028

7. World Health Organization. (2020, May 13). Smallpox. Retrieved August 31, 2020, from https://www.who.int/csr/disease/smallpox/en/

8. Chaib, F. (2019, December 13). WHO commemorates the 40th anniversary of smallpox eradication. Retrieved August 31, 2020, from https://www.who.int/news-room/detail/13-12-2019-who-commemorates-the-40th-anniversary-of-smallpox-eradication

9. Barker, C., & Markmann, J. (2013, April 01). Historical overview of transplantation. Retrieved August 31, 2020, from https://www.ncbi.nlm.nih.gov/pmc/articles/PMC3684003/

10. WEDU. (1998). A Science Odyssey: People and Discoveries: First successful kidney transplant performed. Retrieved August 5, 2020, from http://www.pbs.org/wgbh/aso/databank/entries/dm54ki.html

11. Powell, A. (2019, March 18). A transplant makes history. Retrieved August 5, 2020, from https://news.harvard.edu/gazette/story/2011/09/a-transplant-makes-history/

12. Murray, J. (1990). Nobel Prize Lecture: The First Successful Transplant in Man. Retrieved August 31, 2020, from https://web.stanford.edu/dept/HPST/transplant/html/murray.html

13. United Network for Organ Sharing. (2020, August 25). Organ transplant trends: More transplants than ever. Retrieved March 1, 2021 from https://unos.org/data/transplant-trends/

14. Ahmed, N. (2005, October 31). 23 years of the discovery of Helicobacter pylori: Is the debate over? Retrieved September 01, 2020, from https://www.ncbi.nlm.nih.gov/pmc/articles/PMC1283743/

15. Graham, D. (2014, May 14). History of Helicobacter pylori, duodenal ulcer, gastric ulcer and gastric cancer. Retrieved September 01, 2020, from https://www.ncbi.nlm.nih.gov/pmc/articles/PMC4017034/

16. GI Society: Canadian Society for Intestinal Research. (2020, July 07). Nobel Prize for H. pylori Discovery. Retrieved September 01, 2020, from https://badgut.org/information-centre/a-z-digestive-topics/nobel-prize-for-h-pylori-discovery/

Chapter 2: Refocus Your Vision and Reinvent Your Perspective

17. Wikipedia.com. (2020, October 30). Benjamin Franklin. Retrieved November 03, 2020, from https://en.wikipedia.org/wiki/Benjamin_Franklin

18. Courney, S. (2018, September 27). Benjamin Frankling: American visionary. Retrieved November 03, 2020, from https://www.courant.com/news/connecticut/hc-xpm-2002-09-29-0209290474-story.html

19. Courney, S. (2018, September 27). BENJAMIN FRANKLIN: AMERICAN VISIONARY. Retrieved November 03, 2020, from https://www.courant.com/news/connecticut/hc-xpm-2002-09-29-0209290474-story.html

20. Winstonchurchill.org. (2017, April 13). Churchill: Leader and Statesman. Retrieved November 03, 2020, from https://winstonchurchill.org/the-life-of-churchill/life/churchill-leader-and-statesman/

21. Biography.com Editors. (2020, April 27). Winston Churchill Biography. Retrieved November 03, 2020, from https://www.biography.com/political-figure/winston-churchill

22. Wikimedia. (2020, September 24). British statesman, army officer, and writer (1874–1965). Retrieved November 03, 2020, from https://en.wikiquote.org/wiki/Winston_Churchill

23. AN, S. (2017, December 16). Elon Musk- The Complete Journey of a Visionary Entrepreneur [Bonus Free Videos]. Retrieved November 10, 2020, from https://www.shoutmeloud.com/elon-musk.html

Chapter 3: Redevelop a Growth Mindset and Restructure Your Neurons

24. Popova, M. (2020, February 16). Fixed vs. growth: The two Basic mindsets that shape our lives. Retrieved March 12, 2021, from https://www.brainpickings.org/2014/01/29/carol-dweck-mindset/

25. Sarrasin, J., Nenciovici, L., Foisy, L., Allaire-Duquette, G., Riopel, M., & Masson, S. (2018, July 29). Effects of teaching the concept of neuroplasticity to induce a growth mindset on motivation, achievement, and brain activity: A meta-analysis. Retrieved November 25,

2020, from Brainsworks. (2020). What is Neuroplasticity? Retrieved November 25, 2020, from https://brainworksneurotherapy.com/what-neuroplasticity

26. Wikipedia. (2020, November 24). Neuroplasticity. Retrieved November 25, 2020, from https://en.wikipedia.org/wiki/Neuroplasticity

27. Rossall School. (2018, September 27). Neuroplasticity and Growth Mindsets. Retrieved November 25, 2020, from https://www.rossall.org.uk/neuroplasticity-and-growth-mindsets/

28. Ng, B. (2018, January 26). The Neuroscience of Growth Mindset and Intrinsic Motivation. Retrieved November 25, 2020, from https://www.ncbi.nlm.nih.gov/pmc/articles/PMC5836039/

29. Shaffer, J. (2016, July 26). Neuroplasticity and Clinical Practice: Building Brain Power for Health. Retrieved November 25, 2020, from https://www.ncbi.nlm.nih.gov/pmc/articles/PMC4960264/

30. Garg, R. (2014, January 09). Mindfulness meditation: A mental workout to benefit the brain. Retrieved November 25, 2020, from http://sitn.hms.harvard.edu/flash/2013/mindfulness-meditation-a-mental-workout-to-benefit-the-brain/

31. Lazar, S., Kerr, C., Wasserman, R., Gray, J., Greve, D., Treadway, M., . . . Fischl, B. (2005, November 28). Meditation experience is associated with increased cortical thickness. Retrieved November 25, 2020, from https://www.ncbi.nlm.nih.gov/pmc/articles/PMC1361002/

32. Budde, H., Wegner, M., Soya, H., Voelcker-Rehage, C., & McMorris, T. (2016, October 13). Neuroscience of Exercise: Neuroplasticity and Its Behavioral Consequences. Retrieved November 25, 2020, from https://www.hindawi.com/journals/np/2016/3643879/

33. Erickson, K., Leckie, R., & Weinstein, A. (2014, September). Physical activity, fitness, and gray matter volume. Retrieved November 25, 2020, from https://www.ncbi.nlm.nih.gov/pmc/articles/PMC4094356/

34. Erickson, K., Voss, M., Prakash, R., Basak, C., Szabo, A., Chaddock, L., . . . Kramer, A. (2011, February 15). Exercise training increases size of hippocampus and improves memory. Retrieved November 25, 2020, from https://www.pnas.org/content/108/7/3017?sid=82ba1542-3753-49b2-a1e0-2b16c0b8686b

35. Lin, T., Tsai, S., & Kuo, Y. (2018, December 12). Physical Exercise Enhances Neuroplasticity and Delays Alzheimer's Disease. Retrieved November 25, 2020, from https://www.ncbi.nlm.nih.gov/pmc/articles/PMC6296269/

36. Guzman-Marin, R., & McGinty, D. (2016, July 28). Sleep deprivation suppresses adult neurogenesis: Clues to the role of sleep in brain plasticity. Retrieved November 25, 2020, from https://link.springer.com/article/10.1111/j.1479-8425.2006.00203.x

37. Mueller, A., McGinty, D., & Mistlberger, R. (2015). Sleep and adult neurogenesis: Implications for cognition and mood. Retrieved November 26, 2020, from https://pubmed.ncbi.nlm.nih.gov/24218292/

38. Smith, M., Robinson, L., & Segal, R. (2020, October). How to Sleep Better. Retrieved November 26, 2020, from https://www.helpguide.org/articles/sleep/getting-better-sleep.htm

Chapter 4: Burnout Counselor

39. Smith, M., Segal, J., & Robinson, L. (2020, October). Burnout Prevention and Treatment. Retrieved October 29, 2020, from https://www.helpguide.org/articles/stress/burnout-prevention-and-recovery.htm

40. Imms, A. (2020). The Burnout Project. Retrieved October 30, 2020, from https://theburnoutproject.com.au/

41. World Health Organization. (2019, May 28). Burn-out an "occupational phenomenon": International Classification of Diseases. Retrieved October 30, 2020, from https://www.who.int/mental_health/evidence/burn-out/en/

42. Imms, A. (2020, October 17). Personal interview [Video interview].

43. Stevenson, M. (2020, January 17). Employee Burnout Statistics You Need to Know. Retrieved October 30, 2020, from https://www.hrexchangenetwork.com/employee-engagement/news/employee-burnout-statistics-you-need-to-know

44. Fisher, Jen. (2020, April 24). Workplace Burnout Survey: Deloitte US. Retrieved October 30, 2020, from https://www2.deloitte.com/us/en/pages/about-deloitte/articles/burnout-survey.html

45. Kane, L. (2020, January 15). Medscape National Physician Burnout & Suicide Report 2020: The Generational Divide. Retrieved October 30, 2020, from https://www.medscape.com/slideshow/2020-lifestyle-burnout-6012460

46. Yasgur, B. (2019, January 28). Challenging Stigma: Should Psychiatrists Disclose Their Own Mental Illness? Retrieved October 30, 2020, from https://www.psychiatryadvisor.com/home/topics/mood-disorders/depressive-disorder/challenging-stigma-should-psychiatrists-disclose-their-own-mental-illness/

Chapter 5: Certified Life Coach and Cancer Coach

47. International Coach Federation. (2020). About International Coach Federation. Retrieved November 04, 2020, from https://coachfederation.org/about

48. International Coach Federation. (2016). 2016 ICF Global Coaching Study. Retrieved November 04, 2020, from https://coachfederation.org/app/uploads/2017/12/2016ICFGlobalCoachingStudy_ExecutiveSummary-2.pdf

49. Uță, I. (2020, September 10). Business Coaching Industry to top $15 billion in 2019. Retrieved November 05, 2020, from https://brandminds.live/business-coaching-industry-to-top-15-billion-in-2019/

50. Sherpa Consulting. (2020). Executive Coaching Survey Summary. Retrieved November 05, 2020, from https://www.sherpacoaching.com/pdf_files/2020_Executive_Coaching_Survey_EXECUTIVE_SUMMARY_FINAL.pdf

51. R., A. (2020, October 26). Personal interview [Video interview].

52. International Association of Coaching. (2020, September 06). About International Association of Coaching. Retrieved November 05, 2020, from https://certifiedcoach.org/about/

53. Moser, S. (2020, May 26). How Entrepreneurs Can Join Europe's Booming Coaching Industry. Retrieved January 11, 2021, from https://www.entrepreneur.com/article/348857

Chapter 6: Clinical Content Manager

54. Glassdoor.com. (2020). Salary: Clinical Content Manager. Retrieved November 10, 2020, from https://www.glassdoor.com/Salaries/clinical-content-manager-salary-SRCH_KO0,24.htm

55. Indradjaja, P. (2020, November 04). Personal Interview [Video interview].

56. Builtinnyc.com. (2020, November). Medical Content Manager - Ro: Built In NYC. Retrieved November 10, 2020, from https://www.builtinnyc.com/job/content/medical-content-manager/77870

57. Formstack. (2020). Top 5 Healthcare Marketing Trends for the Digital Age. Retrieved November 20, 2020, from https://www.formstack.com/resources/guide-healthcare-marketing-trends

58. ReferralMD. (2020, June 10). 24 Outstanding Statistics on How Social Media has Impacted Health Care. Retrieved November 20, 2020, from https://getreferralmd.com/2013/09/healthcare-social-media-statistics/

59. Teicher, J. (2020, October 08). 5 Content Marketing Trends Transforming the Healthcare Industry. Retrieved November 20, 2020, from https://contently.com/2020/06/11/healthcare-content-marketing-report/

Chapter 7: Entrepreneur

60. Hayes, A. (2020, September 16). What You Should Know About Entrepreneurs. Retrieved January 06, 2021, from https://www.investopedia.com/terms/e/entrepreneur.asp

61. Vu, T. (2020, October 21). Personal Interview [Video interview].

62. Freedman, M. (2020, April 22). What Does It Mean to Be an Entrepreneur? Retrieved January 06, 2021, from https://www.businessnewsdaily.com/7275-entrepreneurship-defined.html

63. Lin, Y. (2020, December 17). 10 Entrepreneur Stats That You Need To Know in 2021 [INFOGRAPHIC]. Retrieved January 06, 2021, from https://www.oberlo.com/blog/entrepreneur-statistics

64. Hayes, A. (2020, December 22). Business Plans: The Ins and Outs. Retrieved January 06, 2021, from https://www.investopedia.com/terms/b/business-plan.asp

Chapter 8: Global Health Advisor

65. ZipRecruiter.com. (2020). Global Health Consultant Annual Salary. Retrieved December 05, 2020, from https://www.ziprecruiter.com/Salaries/Global-Health-Consultant-Salary

66. MacArthur, S. (2020). Top 10 International Public Health Careers. Retrieved December 06, 2020, from https://www.mphonline.org/best-international-public-health-jobs/

67. Lucero-Prisno, D. (2020, September 19). Personal Interview [Video interview].

68. Healthcare Administration Degree Programs. (2020). What Is A Public Health Advisor? Retrieved December 06, 2020, from https://www.healthcare-administration-degree.net/faq/what-is-a-public-health-advisor/

69. USAIDS. (2015, August). Survey of Major Employers of Global Health Personnel - Executive Summary. Retrieved December 08, 2020, from https://sph.unc.edu/files/2015/10/executive-summary-survey-global-health-career.pdf

70. Keralis, J., Riggin-Pathak, B., Majeski, T., Pathak, B., Foggia, J., Cullinen, K., . . . West, H. (2018). Mapping the global health employment market: An analysis of global health jobs. *BMC Public Health* **18**, 293 (2018). Retrieved December 08, 2020, from https://bmcpublichealth.biomedcentral.com/articles/10.1186/s12889-018-5195-1

71. Myers, D. (2020, June 01). Hang on, New Public Health Grads: Strong Long-Term Outlook for Jobs. Retrieved December 09, 2020, from https://www.globalhealthnow.org/2020-06/hang-new-public-health-grads-strong-long-term-outlook-jobs

Chapter 9: Health Informatics Specialist

72. Zippia.com. (2020, October 02). Here's How To Become A Health Informatics Specialist In 2020. Retrieved October 29, 2020, from https://www.zippia.com/health-informatics-specialist-jobs/

73. USF Health. (2020). Health Informatics. Retrieved October 26, 2020, from https://www.usfhealthonline.com/resources/key-concepts/what-is-health-informatics/

74. Wikipedia. (2020, October 19). Health informatics. Retrieved October 26, 2020, from https://en.wikipedia.org/wiki/Health_informatics

75. Healthcare Management Degree Guide. (2020). What Exactly is "Health Informatics"? Retrieved October 27, 2020, from https://www.healthcare-management-degree.net/faq/what-exactly-is-health-informatics/

76. Mack, J. (2020, March 31). Health Informatics Explained. Retrieved October 27, 2020, from https://onlinedegrees.sandiego.edu/what-is-health-informatics/

77. Sulaiman, I. (2020, October 11). Personal Interview [Video interview].

78. OCR. (2017, June 16). HITECH Act Enforcement Interim Final Rule. Retrieved November 20, 2020, from https://www.hhs.gov/hipaa/for-professionals/special-topics/hitech-act-enforcement-interim-final-rule/index.html

79. Kierkegaard, P. (2011, September 16). Electronic health record: Wiring Europe's healthcare. Retrieved November 20, 2020, from https://www.sciencedirect.com/science/article/abs/pii/S0267364911001257?via=ihub

80. UIC Online. (2020, July 09). Clinical Informatics Specialist Career Spotlight: UIC Online. Retrieved October 29, 2020, from https://healthinformatics.uic.edu/blog/career-spotlight-clinical-informatics-specialist/

Chapter 10: Health Insurance Advisor

81. US Bureau of Labor Statistics. (2020, September 01). Insurance Sales Agents : Occupational Outlook Handbook. Retrieved October 19, 2020, from https://www.bls.gov/ooh/sales/insurance-sales-agents.htm

82. Kennelly, R. (2020). What Is a Health Insurance Broker? Retrieved October 14, 2020, from https://help.ihealthagents.com/hc/en-us/articles/360007446474-What-Is-a-Health-Insurance-Broker-

83. Ali, N. (2020, September 10). Personal Interview [Video interview].

84. Kaplan Financial Education. (2020, July 31). 5 Reasons Insurance Sales is a Good Career. Retrieved October 19, 2020, from https://www.kaplanfinancial.com/resources/getting-started/5-reasons-insurance-sales-is-a-good-career

85. Insureon, Small Business Blog. (2020, May 14). 5 Rock-Solid Reasons to Choose a Career in Insurance. Retrieved October 19, 2020, from https://www.insureon.com/blog/why-choose-an-insurance-career

Chapter 11: Home Health Care Continuum

86. ZipRecruiter.com. (2020). Home Health Registered Nurse Annual Salary. Retrieved November 21, 2020, from https://www.ziprecruiter.com/Salaries/Home-Health-Registered-Nurse-Salary

87. Grand View Research. (2020, May). Home Healthcare Market Size, Growth Report, 2020-2027. Retrieved November 07, 2020, from https://www.grandviewresearch.com/industry-analysis/home-healthcare-industry

88. Cunanan, C. (2020, November 03). Personal Interview [Video interview].

89. Elliot, B. (2014, December). Nursing 2020: Considering home healthcare nursing? Retrieved November 05, 2020, from https://www.nursingcenter.com/journalarticle?Article_ID=2651897

90. Betterteam.com. (2020). Clinical Supervisor Job Description. Retrieved November 07, 2020, from https://www.betterteam.com/clinical-supervisor-job-description

91. Simione Healthcare Consultants. (2020). Inside the Clinical Manager Role: Leadership for Exceptional Team-Based Care. Retrieved November 06, 2020, from https://www.simione.com/application/files/7715/1214/8309/inside-the-clinical-manager-role.pdf

Chapter 12: Medical Educator

92. Glassdoor.com. (2020). Medical Educator. Retrieved December 04, 2020, from https://www.glassdoor.com/Salaries/medical-educator-salary-SRCH_KO0,16.htm

93. Stewart, R. (2020, October 22). Personal Interview [Video interview].

94. Bls.gov. (2020, September 01). Health Educators and Community Health Workers : Occupational Outlook Handbook. Retrieved December 04, 2020, from https://www.bls.gov/ooh/community-and-social-service/health-educators.htm

95. Bartle, Emma, and Jill Thistlethwaite . "Becoming a Medical Educator: Motivation, Socialisation and Navigation." *BMC Medical Education*, BioMed Central, 21 May 2014, bmcmededuc.biomedcentral.com/articles/10.1186/1472-6920-14-110.

96. AMEE. (2020). AMEE: An International Association for Medical Education. Retrieved December 13, 2020, from https://amee.org/home

97. Academy of Medical Educators. (2014, October). Professional Standards for medical, dental and veterinary educators. Retrieved October 31, 2020, from https://www.medicaleducators.org/write/MediaManager/AOME_Professional_Standards_2014.pdf

98. CPMEC. (2020). Confederation of Postgraduate Medical Education Councils (CPMEC). Retrieved December 13, 2020, from http://www.cpmec.org.au/

99. Wikipedia. (2020, October 14). Academic tenure. Retrieved December 05, 2020, from https://en.wikipedia.org/wiki/Academic_tenure

100. Raghavan, M., Martin, B., Ripstein, I., & Sandham, D. (2015, August 18). Managing Growth in Medical Education: International Association of Medical Science Educators. Retrieved October 31, 2020, from http://www.iamse.org/mse-article/managing-growth-in-medical-education/

101. Han, E., Yeo, S., Kim, M., Lee, Y., Park, K., & Roh, H. (2019, December 11). Medical education trends for future physicians in the era of advanced technology and artificial intelligence: An integrative review. Retrieved October 31, 2020, from https://bmcmededuc.biomedcentral.com/articles/10.1186/s12909-019-1891-5

102. Jakubek, K. (2019, April 09). AMA expansion of national effort creating medical school of the future. Retrieved October 31, 2020, from https://www.ama-assn.org/press-center/press-releases/ama-expansion-national-effort-creating-medical-school-future

Chapter 13: Medical Reviewer

103. Study.com. (2019, September 15). Medical Reviewer: Job Description, Duties and Requirements. Retrieved September 02, 2020, from https://study.com/articles/Medical_Reviewer_Job_Description_Duties_and_Requirements.html

104. Moawad, H. (2020). Medical Review Companies. Retrieved November 21, 2020, from http://www.nonclinicaldoctors.com/medical-review-companies.html

105. ZipRecruiter.com. (2020, August 26). Medical Reviewer Annual Salary ($71,298 Avg: Aug 2020). Retrieved September 02, 2020, from https://www.ziprecruiter.com/Salaries/Medical-Reviewer-Salary

106. Asencio, L. (2020, September 1). Personal Interview [Video interview].

107. Prescient & Strategic Intelligence Private Limited. (2020). Market Research. Retrieved November 21, 2020, from https://www.reportlinker.com/p05932750/U-S-Medical-Peer-External-Physician-Review-Services-Market.html?utm_source=GNW

108. LeverageRx. (2019). 2019 medical malpractice payout report [infographic]. Retrieved March 12, 2021, from https://www.leveragerx.com/malpractice-insurance/2019-medical-malpractice-report/

109. Cappellino, A. (2020, June 25). Medical malpractice PAYOUT report for 2018. Retrieved March 12, 2021, from https://www.expertinstitute.com/resources/insights/medical-malpractice-payout-report-for-2018/

Chapter 14: Medical Science Liaison

110. Indeed.com. (2020, October 12). What Does a Medical Science Liaison Do? The Role, Duties, Salary and How To Become One. Retrieved October 20, 2020, from https://www.indeed.com/career-advice/finding-a-job/medical-science-liaison

111. Gani, F. (2020). Becoming a Medical Science Liaison - Jobs, Salary & Education. Retrieved October 20, 2020, from https://www.healthcaredegree.com/administration/medical-science-liaison

112. Explorehealthcareers.org. (2018, February 07). Medical Science Liaison. Retrieved October 20, 2020, from https://explorehealthcareers.org/career/pharmacology/medical-science-liaison/

113. MSL Society. (2020, July 20). What is a Medical Science Liaison (MSL)? Retrieved October 20, 2020, from https://www.themsls.org/what-is-an-msl/

114. Madrigal-Iberri, C. (2020, October 12). Personal Interview [Video interview].

115. BCMAs. (2020). Medical Science Liaison Training. Retrieved November 22, 2020, from https://www.medicalaffairsspecialist.org/medical-science-liaison-msl-training/

116. Parker, P. (2019, November 27). Medical Science Liaison Jobs: The Best-Kept Secret in the Life Sciences Industry. Retrieved November 21, 2020, from https://www.biospace.com/article/medical-science-liaison-jobs-the-best-kept-secret-in-the-life-sciences-industry/

117. Yuri. (2020, August 04). Is A Medical Science Liaison (MSL) Job Right For You? Retrieved November 22, 2020, from https://cheekyscientist.com/how-to-know-if-a-medical-science-liaison-job-is-right-for-you/

Chapter 15: Medical Scientist

118. Bls.gov, A. (2020, September 01). Medical Scientists: Occupational Outlook Handbook. Retrieved November 19, 2020, from https://www.bls.gov/ooh/life-physical-and-social-science/medical-scientists.htm

119. Majeed, N. (2020, October 14). Personal Interview [Video interview].

120. Israr, S., Hayat, A., Ahmad, T., Majeed, N., Naqvi, S., & Tehseen, S. (2020, June). Comparison of Procalcitonin and Hematological Ratios in Cord Blood as Early Predictive Marker of Neonatal Sepsis. Retrieved October 28, 2020, from https://www.pafmj.org/index.php/PAFMJ/article/view/4670

121. Hayat, A., Jaffar, S., Majeed, N., Abbas, S., Asghar, J., & Tayyab, N. (2020, July). Association of Liver Function Derangements with Disease Severity in COVID-19 Patients. Retrieved October 28, 2020, from https://www.pafmj.org/index.php/PAFMJ/article/view/4889

122. Du, X., Ou, Y., Xu, S., He, B., Luo, W., & Jiang, D. (2020, May 19). Comparison of three different bone GRAFT methods for single Segment lumbar TUBERCULOSIS: A retrospective SINGLE-CENTER cohort study. Retrieved October 28, 2020, from https://www.sciencedirect.com/science/article/pii/S1743919120304222

Chapter 16: Pharmaceutical Ethics and Compliance Continuum

123. Salary.com. (2020, November 25). Ethics and Compliance Officer Salary. Retrieved December 12, 2020, from https://www.salary.com/research/salary/alternate/ethics-and-compliance-officer-salary

124. Khor, SK. (2020, October 22). Personal interview [Video interview].

125. O'Neill-Mathias, A. (2017, November 21). Interview: Anne O'Neill-Mathias, Head of Ethics and Compliance, Roche Pharmaceuticals. Retrieved December 12, 2020, from https://www.mendeley.com/careers/news/careers-jobs-field/interview-anne-oneill-mathias-head-ethics-and-compliance-roche

126. Khan, R. (2020, November 10). Work From Anywhere Trend Intensifying Ethics, And Compliance Issues. Retrieved December 13, 2020, from https://www.forbes.com/sites/roomykhan/2020/11/06/work-from-anywhere-trend-intensifying-ethics-and-compliance-issues/?sh=4173d15f2f38

127. Volkov, M. (2020, January 14). Ethics and Compliance Trends and Predictions for 2020. Retrieved December 13, 2020, from https://www.jdsupra.com/legalnews/ethics-and-compliance-trends-and-59223/

Chapter 17: Planetary Doctor

128. Wikipedia. (2020, December 12). Planetary health. Retrieved December 15, 2020, from https://en.wikipedia.org/wiki/Planetary_health

129. Webb, K. (2019, April 22). The planet is the patient now: How doctors and nurses are the front-line solution to climate change. Retrieved December 15, 2020, from https://www.salon.com/2019/04/21/the-planet-is-the-patient-now-how-doctors-and-nurses-are-the-front-line-solution-to-climate-change/

130. Capon, A., Talley, N., & Horton, R. (2018). Planetary health: What is it and what should doctors do? Retrieved December 15, 2020, from https://www.mja.com.au/system/files/issues/208_07/10.5694mja18.00219.pdf

131. Guinto, R. (2020, September 12). Personal interview [Video interview].

132. Clinicians for Planetary Health (C4PH). (2020). Planetary Health Alliance, Clinicians for Planetary Health. Retrieved December 15, 2020, from https://www.planetaryhealthalliance.org/clinicians-for-planetary-health

133. Panoramaglobal. (2017, September). Panorama Perspective: Conversations on Planetary Health. Retrieved December 19, 2020, from https://www.rockefellerfoundation.org/wp-content/uploads/Planetary-Health-101-Information-and-Resources.pdf

134. Wikipedia. (2020, December 10). Planetary boundaries. Retrieved December 18, 2020, from https://en.wikipedia.org/wiki/Planetary_boundaries

Chapter 18: Professor

135. Glassdoor.com. (2020). Professor Salaries. Retrieved December 20, 2020, from https://www.glassdoor.com/Salaries/professor-salary-SRCH_KO0,9.htm

136. Bureau of Labor Statistics. (2020, September 01). Postsecondary Teachers: Occupational Outlook Handbook. Retrieved December 20, 2020, from https://www.bls.gov/ooh/education-training-and-library/postsecondary-teachers.htm

137. Wikipedia. (2020, December 19). Professor. Retrieved December 20, 2020, from https://en.wikipedia.org/wiki/Professor

138. CareerExplorer. (2019, November 14). What does a professor do? Retrieved December 21, 2020, from https://www.careerexplorer.com/careers/professor/

139. Hartigan-Go, K. (2020, September 12). Personal interview [Video interview].

140. Wikipedia. (2020, October 14). Academic tenure. Retrieved December 05, 2020, from https://en.wikipedia.org/wiki/Academic_tenure

141. Raise Labs. (2020). Postsecondary Teachers: Salary, career path, job outlook, education and more. Retrieved January 04, 2021, from https://www.raise.me/careers/education-training-and-library/postsecondary-teachers

142. Spear, E. (2019, December 18). 10 Trends in Higher Education to Watch in 2020. Retrieved January 04, 2021, from https://precisioncampus.com/blog/trends-higher-education/

143. Hatcher, J. (2020, January). 4 Emerging Trends That Will Create Opportunities for Universities in 2020. Retrieved January 04, 2021, from https://www.insidehighered.com/sponsored/4-emerging-trends-will-create-opportunities-universities-2020

Chapter 19: Quality Coordinator

144. Zippia.com. (2020, October 02). Here's How To Become A Quality Coordinator In 2020. Retrieved October 23, 2020, from https://www.zippia.com/quality-coordinator-jobs/

145. Learn.org, A. (2020). Quality Assurance Manager. Retrieved November 23, 2020, from https://learn.org/articles/Quality_Assurance_Manager_Job_Duties_Career_Outlook_and_Education_Prerequisites.html

146. El Bassit, G. (2020, September 15). Personal interview [Video interview].

147. Betterteam.com. (2019, July 12). Quality Coordinator Job Description. Retrieved October 23, 2020, from https://www.betterteam.com/quality-coordinator-job-description

148. Relationships Australia. (2017, January). Position Description for Quality Coordinator. Retrieved October 22, 2020, from https://www.raq.org.au/sites/raq/files/Quality%20Coordinator.pdf

Chapter 20: Ship Physician

149. Shopov, I. (2019). Cruise Ship Jobs - Doctor / Physician Jobs. Retrieved December 30, 2020, from https://www.cruiseshipjob.com/doctor-jobs.html

150. C. Gonzalez (personal communication, December 30, 2020).

151. Cruise.jobs, A. (2020). Significance of Epaulettes worn by Cruise Ship Staff. Retrieved December 31, 2020, from https://cruise.jobs/stripes/

152. Fawcett, C. (2018, May 21). What to do if you want to be a cruise ship doctor. Retrieved December 31, 2020, from https://www.kevinmd.com/blog/2018/05/what-to-do-if-you-want-to-be-a-cruise-ship-doctor.html

153. Giese, M. (2020, July 23). COVID-19 impacts on global cruise industry. Retrieved January 03, 2021, from https://home.kpmg/xx/en/blogs/home/posts/2020/07/covid-19-impacts-on-global-cruise-industry.html

154. Norton, T. (2020, December 23). An Outlook on the State of the Cruise Industry for 2021. Retrieved January 03, 2021, from https://www.travelpulse.com/gallery/cruise/an-outlook-on-the-state-of-the-cruise-industry-for-2021.html?image=5

Chapter 21: Sharpen Your Knowledge

155. Pathak, P. (2015, March 18). 13 life lessons from Eagles. Retrieved December 03, 2020, from https://www.speakingtree.in/allslides/13-life-lessons-from-eagles/263791

156. Wikipedia.com. (2020, November 30). Knowledge. Retrieved December 03, 2020, from https://en.wikipedia.org/wiki/Knowledge

157. Temsen, R., & Whalen, R. (2019, January 15). Why Is Reading Important? The 11 Benefits Of Books. Retrieved December 03, 2020, from https://www.bestpracticeinhr.com/why-is-reading-important-the-11-benefits-of-books/

158. Edx.org (2020). Deliver inspiring learning experiences on any scale. Retrieved December 03, 2020, from https://open.edx.org/

159. Coursera.org. (2020, December 01). About. Retrieved December 03, 2020, from https://about.coursera.org/

160. Udemy.com. (2020, September 09). Learn about Udemy culture, mission, and careers: About Us. Retrieved December 03, 2020, from https://about.udemy.com/

Chapter 22 – Select Your Mentors

161. Grimmer, F. (2016, June 02). Accelerate Your Career: The Power of Mentorship. Retrieved November 30, 2020, from https://horizonone.com.au/2013/09/accelerate-your-career-the-power-of-mentorship/

162. Bidwell, L. (2020). Why Mentors Matter: A Summary of 30 Years of Research. Retrieved November 30, 2020, from https://www.sap.com/insights/hr/why-mentors-matter.html

163. Stringer, H. (2016, June). The life-changing power of mentors. Retrieved November 30, 2020, from https://www.apa.org/monitor/2016/06/mentors

164. Allen, T., Eby, L., Poteet, M., Lentz, E., & Lima, L. (2004). APA PsycNet. Retrieved November 30, 2020, from https://content.apa.org/doiLanding?doi=10.1037%2F0021-9010.89.1.127

165. Grimmer, F. (2016, June 02). Accelerate Your Career: The Power of Mentorship. Retrieved December 02, 2020, from https://horizonone.com.au/2013/09/accelerate-your-career-the-power-of-mentorship/

166. Zhao, P. (2018, December 06). The Power of Mentorship. Retrieved December 02, 2020, from https://medium.com/@ppz12985/the-power-of-mentorship-965a86cfc40

167. Horoszowski, M. (2020). How to Build a Great Relationship with a Mentor. Retrieved December 02, 2020, from https://hbr-org.cdn.ampproject.org/c/s/hbr.org/amp/2020/01/how-to-build-a-great-relationship-with-a-mentor

Chapter 23: Strengthen Your Network

168. Jason, A. (2020, April 13). Amazing Eagle Facts, Principles, and Lessons That Will Change Your Life. Retrieved December 02, 2020, from https://wealthanize.com/eagle-facts-life-principles-lessons/

169. Bonds-Raacke, J., Raacke, J., & Elliott2017, S. (2017, January). Should I be networking? Exploring the importance of networking for students. Retrieved December 02, 2020, from https://www.apa.org/ed/precollege/psn/2017/01/importance-networking

170. Hurtado, J. (2020, October 27). The Importance of Networking: Why Networking Skills are Necessary. Retrieved December 03, 2020, from https://capital-placement.com/blog/the-importance-of-networking/

171. LinkedIn Corporate, A. (2017, June 22). Eighty-percent of professionals consider networking important to career success. Retrieved December 03, 2020, from https://news.linkedin.com/2017/6/eighty-percent-of-professionals-consider-networking-important-to-career-success

172. Page, M. (2018, May 11). Top 11 benefits of networking. Retrieved December 03, 2020, from https://www.michaelpage.com.au/advice/career-advice/career-progression/benefits-networking

Testimonials (continued)

"Nicole is a leader who spearheaded various projects as a Clinical Manager, Clinical Specialist, Director of Performance Outcomes, and Director of Managed Care and Business Development. She led a team to improve organizational processes and maximize opportunities in revenue cycle management. Nicole is a transformational leader who is charismatic and articulate. She has high moral standards and ethical behavior. She will walk the talk."

Mila Smith
Healthcare Consultant

"I first met Nicole when we were medical students in the Philippines. We studied in different schools on separate islands, but somehow her wit and charm drew me to work with her on a research project that we presented at an international conference. The topic was about preventative healthcare practices of seafarers, a topic close to her heart, as her hometown of Iloilo has produced many of the world's commercial seafarers. Raised in a Filipino-American home, Nicole is passionate about bringing attention to the issues from her unique cultural upbringing, making them relatable to a broader audience as if asking them to visit her home. It comes as no surprise that Nicole wrote this book. She is likewise introducing multiple worlds to an audience who only knew a few rigid paths to professional life. We doctors are so concerned about "medicine" that we forget about the rapidly changing world outside, and that this world has an increasing niche for us. Nicole is inviting us in, to visit and see for ourselves. Don't mind if I do."

Dr. Michael Pineda
Neurologist

"I've known Nicole for more than a decade now. We met back in 2009 when we were first partnered as exchange students in Kanazawa, Japan under AMSA. She has always been amiable, caring, and a delightful person to be with. Her positive demeanor and outlook, coupled with her enthusiasm in helping colleagues in AMSA and beyond the organization, makes her a valuable asset in the community.

I have always admired Nicole for her industry, perseverance, and determination in reaching her goals and dreams. In whatever Nicole pursues, she always does it to the best of her capabilities."

Dr. Joanna Marie D. Choa-Go
Pediatric Radiologist

"I've known Nicole for years now, since we met in medical school and in AMSA International, which she led. She brought a fresh perspective on student/club governance, community activities, and introduced us to a wider (international) community. She's always been the one to break out of the mold, but then she always finds her niche and shines through. I'm always proud, always."

Dr. Melinessa Encarnacion Youngblood
ER Concierge

"It was election day for the Asian Medical Students Association—Philippines, mid-year 2011, and I was sitting in a corner of a room full of passionate medical students from different universities. Nicole nominated me as Treasurer and I won. That is when my aspiration to become a passionate and contributory medical student started. Thank you so much, Dr. Nicole, for your trust and for being an inspiration to me and to many."

Dr. Erica Tania Davillo
Military Doctor
Armed Forces of the Philippines

"Nicole is a go-getter. Her background in medicine, coupled with her innovation and business acumen, displays her knack for resourcefulness and perseverance. She is someone who knows success is a journey, not a destination."

Alexandra Otero Mahjouri
Research Analyst/Deputy Program Manager
Daybreak LLC, supporting United States Central Command (US CENTCOM)

Acknowledgments

I am sincerely thankful for...

God who brought me wisdom and discernment in what to write, what not to write, and how to express myself through the written word. To God be the glory.

My supportive and loving family (Doc Alex, Doc Mergie, Patrick, Doc Angel, and Doc Jake) who encouraged and motivated me to complete an important item on my bucket list of becoming an author. You helped me weather my doubts and persevere.

Judy Altier, my personal editor, who burned the midnight oil to complete this book. Your expertise and mastery of the English language, especially grammar, tone, and presentation are extremely appreciated and praised. Thank you for being meticulous in helping make my work an even stronger book.

The Ultimate 48 Hour Author team (Natasa, Stu, Vivi, Lendy, Julie, and Nik) for your assistance in making this book a reality. I am thankful for your advice through every stage of publishing.

My interviewees (Dr. Amy Imms, Dr. Anitha R, Dr. Patrick Indradjaja, Dr. Vu Tran, Dr Don Eliseo Lucero-Prisno, Dr. Ismat Mohd Sulaiman, Dr. Noor Afsa Ali, Dr. Cezar Cunanan, Dr. Rebecca Stewart, Dr. Luis Asencio, Dr. Carlos Madrigal-Iberri, Dr. Numan Majeed, Dr. Khor Swee Kheng, Dr. Renzo Guinto, Dr. Kenneth Hartigan-Go, and Dr. Ghattas El Bassit) for sharing your inspiring stories and knowledge. Your experiences will guide countless international medical graduates to successful career transition.

My Asian Medical Student Association Alumni friends (Dr. Joseph Assad, Dr. Yoon-Kyo An, and Dr. Dulce Adoracion) for referring amazing medical doctors who pivoted to alternative careers.

JJ & the Lens for taking my profile picture, editing my interviewees' photographs, and integrating my online videos. Your attention to detail and professionalism is appreciated.

Lastly, my extended family members, friends, and colleagues who cheered me on throughout this process and who continue to support me through my endeavors.

About the Author

Nicole is an experienced health professional with over 12 years of hands-on management experience including operational, technological, and clinical aspects of health care. She earned a Doctor of Medicine degree from West Visayas State University College of Medicine in 2012, a Master of Science in Health Informatics degree from University of South Florida in 2019, and a Bachelor of Science in Family, Youth, and Community Sciences degree with three minors from University of Florida in 2006.

Nicole believes in the power of optimism grounded in actionable strategies. At 30 years old, she broke away from her medical path and shifted through multiple career paths. At 35 years old, she had her breakthrough career moment when she joined the largest FQHC (Federally Qualified Health Center) in Florida, USA as Director of Performance Outcomes for 15 health centers and over 80 multi-specialty clinicians. Currently, she works as a Senior Healthcare Consultant serving large scale healthcare organizations globally.

Nicole has successfully led multiple projects on performance improvements, operating systems implementation, practice and utilization management, and revenue cycle management. Key strengths also include bridging analytics with technology and health care to ensure positive patient outcomes.

Nicole is an avid traveler who has toured 36 countries. She currently lives in Clearwater, Florida with her family and two dogs Odie (a Golden Retriever) and Gambit (a German Shepherd). In her spare time, she loves visiting the Dunedin Causeway in her Honda Ridgeline truck, looking out over the Gulf of Mexico and contemplating her next adventure.

NICOLE GUEVARA
MD, MSHI, CPHIMS

Nicole is an experienced health professional with over 12 years of hands-on management experience including operational, technological, and clinical aspects of health care. She earned a Doctor of Medicine degree from West Visayas State University College of Medicine in 2012, a Master of Science in Health Informatics degree from University of South Florida in 2019, and a Bachelor of Science in Family, Youth, and Community Sciences degree with three minors from University of Florida in 2006.

Nicole juggled multiple jobs until her breakthrough in 2019 as Director of Performance Outcomes for Florida's largest Federally Qualified Health Center. Currently, she works as Senior Healthcare Consultant serving large scale healthcare organizations globally. Her key strengths include bridging analytics with technology and health care to ensure positive patient outcomes.

I can be your next Speaker!
Speaking Topics:

1. **Three steps to redefine your destiny**
   a. Realize your breakthrough
   b. Refocus your vision
   c. Redevelop a growth mindset

2. **Three Tips to get ahead of the competition**
   a. Sharpen your knowledge
   b. Strengthen your network
   c. Select your mentor

3. **From Zero to Hero**
   a. Three steps to career transition
   b. You know what you want, now what?
   c. Rocking your next career

www.breakawaymd.com
@ docnicoleg@gmail.com

16 FREE VIDEOS

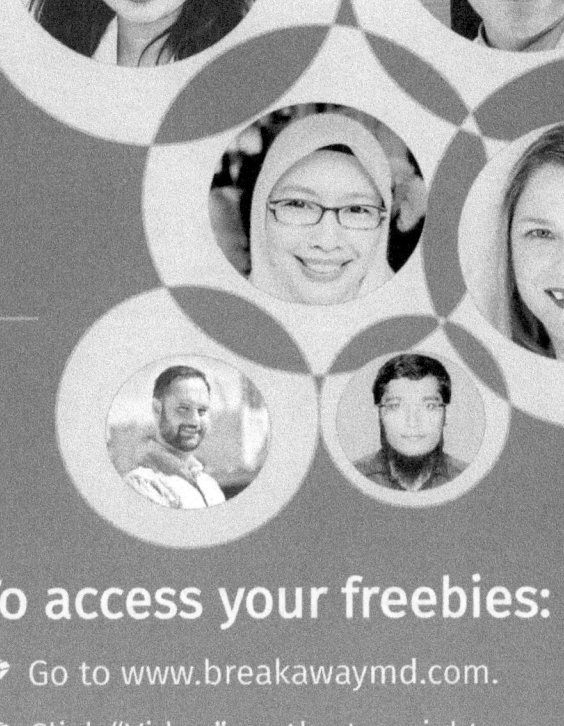

Access ALL 16 interviews in my book as a GIFT to you

These videos detail my interviews with medical professionals across the globe who pivoted to alternative careers.

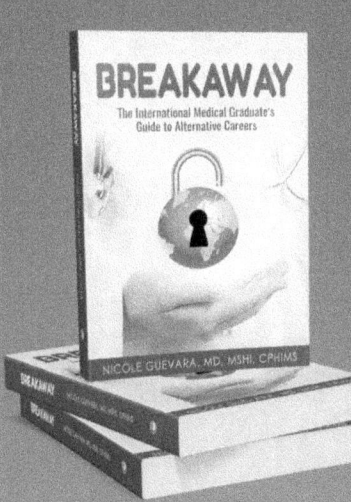

To access your freebies:

- ◆ Go to www.breakawaymd.com.
- ◆ Click "Video" on the top right corner.
- ◆ Enter password: Movingforward
- ◆ Click on the picture of the video you want to watch.

www.breakawaymd.com

I can be your next Podcast Guest:

NICOLE GUEVARA

MD, MSHI, CPHIMS

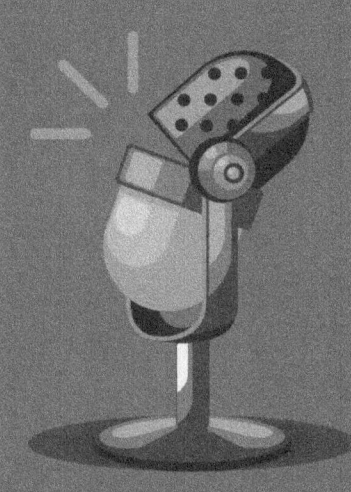

www.breakawaymd.com

Starting fresh after earning my medical degree was not easy. Nicole pivoted through different jobs as Medical Assistant, Home Health Aide, Referral Coordinator, Rehab Counselor, Senior Clinical Coordinator, and Clinical Manager. At 35 years old, she had her breakthrough career moment when she joined the largest Federally Qualified Health Center (FQHC) in Florida, USA as Director of Performance Outcomes for 15 health centers and over 90 multi-specialty clinicians. Nicole has successfully led multiple projects on performance improvements, operating systems implementation, practice and utilization management, and revenue cycle management. Presently, she is doing what she loves leveraging her knowledge and experience as a full-time healthcare consultant serving large scale healthcare organizations globally.

Podcast Topics:

- Breaking away from medicine
- Serenity amidst a chaotic career change
- 3 Tips for getting ahead of the competition